Praise for Juicy Smoot

'We do not consume enough variety of fruits a   smoothies are so much more beneficial than m   health products we buy.

On top of their known contributions, natural fibrous foods provide amino acids, minerals, vitamins and other health-promoting components, many of which are as yet unidentified.'

Professor Robert Nash, Research Director, PhytoQuest Limited

About Professor Nash

Dr. Nash is a global leader in the field of phytochemicals – plant chemicals. He began his research career at the Royal Botanic Gardens Kew.

He has published more than 200 scientific publications and patents.

His focus has been on the discovery of new pharmaceutical compounds from plants and has several compounds in development for diabetes, immune modulation and anti-inflammatory activity.

He was the first winner of the Pierre-Fabre Award of the Phytochemical Society of Europe.

Good Health —

Helen J. Simpson

22.9.2016.

Helen J. Simpson

THE JUICY

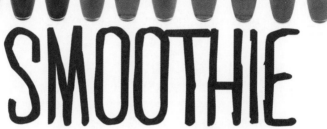

SMOOTHIE

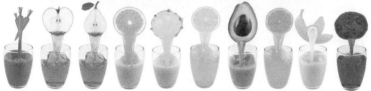

HEALTH BAR

How to juice yourself to permanent
good health and a longer life

foulsham
LONDON • NEW YORK • TORONTO • SYDNEY

W. Foulsham & Co. Ltd
For Foulsham Publishing Ltd
The Old Barrel Store, Drayman's Lane, Marlow, Bucks SL7 2FF

Foulsham books can be found in all good bookshops and direct from
www.foulsham.com

He bringeth forth grass for the cattle: and green herb for the service of men.
Psalm 104:14

ISBN 978-0-572-04630-9

Neither the editors of W. Foulsham & Co. Ltd nor the author nor the publisher take
responsibility for any possible consequences from any treatment, procedure, test,
exercise, action or application of medication or preparation by any person reading or
following the information in this book. The publication of this book does not constitute
the practice of medicine, and this book does not attempt to replace your doctor.

Edited by Helen Jones
Text design Kevin Wade
Cover design Andrew Evans
Typesetting Megan Sheer
Printed in Great Britain by Latimer Trend

Contents

Acknowledgements

I wish to acknowledge the help given to me by the following people: Ann Bagnall of Southover Press; our nephew, soft fruit and apple grower Robert Simpson; pharmacist Robert N. Gardiner; Dr Malcolm Lias; The Royal Society of Chemistry, for permission to use the vitamin and mineral data from their Composition of Food; Dr Tom Sanders and Peter Bazalgette, co-authors of The Food Revolution; John Davidson of the Wholistic Research Company, for his information on buying juicers and for data from his A Harmony of Science and Nature; Brian Clements of the Hippocrates Health Centre, Florida, USA; nutrition scientist Dr Sarah Scheneker of the British Nutrition Foundation; Professor Robert Nash, research director of PhytoQuest Ltd; Liz Kullmann, Registered Dietician and Nutrition Consultant, and Alister Hoda.

Above all, a very special thank you to my editor Helen Jones, for her considerable help in producing this revised and updated version of my book, bringing it further into the twenty-first century.

Introduction

'Foods should be our medicine, and our medicine should be our foods.'

Hippocrates, 359 BC

The connection between diet and health

Most of us aspire to experiencing good health, energy and vitality and staying healthy for many years to come. And yet we don't always give our bodies the best chance of achieving this.

Our everyday diet, for example, is a major contributing factor to our health and well-being but invariably it is not as healthy as it should be. We tend to eat a high proportion of cooked and processed foods and not enough raw fruit and vegetables. Cooking our food destroys much of its vitamin content and creates grievous losses of minerals. Manufacturing processes also strip food of its nutritive value and too often convenience, colour effect and seasoning have become the overriding considerations at the expense of real nourishment.

As a result we suffer from all manner of ailments including migraines, asthma, psoriasis, eczema, arthritis, heart disease, obesity, diabetes and certain cancers. We know that in a health context prevention is always better than cure, so it makes sense to change our diet to a healthier one. Even if we have had a lifetime of unhealthy eating habits, it is not too late to make a difference to our health now.

The unique power of raw fruits and vegetables

We have known instinctively for centuries that a diet containing raw fruits and vegetables, as well as herbs, grasses, sea vegetables, grains and pulses, is essential to the body's health and well-being. Today scientists from all over the world are discovering that naturally occurring nutrients and phytochemicals in living foods can help to fight cancer and other diseases. Raw foods have an extraordinary capacity to promote a high level of health, can cure long-standing illnesses and prevent others from developing.

So, drinking smoothies made from raw fruits and vegetables as part of a sensible, balanced, wholefood diet (high in fibre and low in refined sugars and sodium) is a brilliant way to change old habits and set us on the path to a healthier and happier lifestyle.

Why are home-made smoothies better for us?

Fresh smoothies are bursting with living cells, free from additives and preservatives: canned, bottled and concentrated juices are pasteurised – or irradiated – to increase their shelf life, which destroys some nutrients. In many cases, the manufactured products state that they contain 'added vitamin C' but in this case the vitamin serves only as an antioxidant and not as a nutrient. Shop-bought smoothies also have no restriction on fruit or sugar content and are far inferior in flavour to smoothies made from freshly prepared fruit and vegetables.

How will smoothies improve my health?

By consuming freshly made smoothies on a regular basis, you will not only feel healthier but also acquire more energy and resistance to disease. The restorative powers of fresh fruit smoothies, packed with vitamins, minerals and phytochemicals, and purifying natural acidity, have been called 'body cleansers', and the squeezed fresh vegetable smoothies from sprouts and greens are the 'body restorers', brimming with blood- and bone-building materials.

Freshly made smoothies feed the body with the vitamins and minerals it needs to stay healthy as well as helping to eliminate harmful toxins and accumulated wastes. This leads to better functioning of our organs, stronger bones, muscles and tissues, shiny hair, wrinkle-free skin and firm nails. Consuming smoothies can also actively lower cholesterol and blood pressure, and is a healthy way to support a weight-loss programme.

The recipes in this book are divided into three sections: smoothies to greatly improve health, smoothies to help you lose extra weight and smoothies to help combat specific conditions.

Readers who don't need to lose weight will still benefit from the recipes in that section. Each of the smoothies has been tried out by my editor who has given her unbiased opinion on the flavour, described in the 'taste test'. You can record what you think in the My Verdict box below each recipe.

It is important to note that sole raw juice therapy is not recommended for patients whose immunity has been lowered by chemotherapy or radiotherapy, as all foods must be well cooked and therefore sterilised. Health professionals are concerned that you might be missing out on essential nutrients found in other foods. So consult your doctor regarding your changes in nutrition.

Also fresh fruit juices such as orange juices are now causing concerns with dentists over early tooth decay in children's teeth, caused by the natural fruit sugars, so these drinks should be diluted with at least 50 per cent water. Never put fruit juice into a baby bottle. It must always be given in a cup to a young child.

I began juicing in 2005, and I have continued over the past ten years to make healthy juices and smoothies as part of my everyday lifestyle. Now in my eightieth year, I continue to feel healthy and energetic, and I enjoy encouraging others to do the same. I hope that you will learn from *The Juicy Smoothie Health Bar* that using fresh fruits and vegetables in this form of nutrition will bring you a long and healthy life.

Helen J. Simpson

1. Getting started

'September blow soft 'till the fruits in the loft.'

Thomas Tusser

Equipment

BLENDERS

The main item of equipment you will need to make smoothies is a blender. This can be used for blending bananas, avocados, apricots, yoghurt, milk, water, honey, wheatgerm, seeds and other ingredients with fresh fruit and vegetables to make superb smoothies. High-powered blenders are more expensive but they are the best for achieving a much smoother texture to your smoothie. There are many blenders on the market but the following are my top three recommendations:

Nutri Ninja Pro Blender

My personal favourite, this powerful blender with a 900-watt motor is excellent for making smoothies with a finer consistency. It will even break down frozen fruit and ice cubes. It comes with a range of containers with lids for transporting your drinks. It has a one-year guarantee.

NutriBullet 900

The NutriBullet also has a 900-watt motor and is capable of cutting up nuts and seeds as easily as fruit and vegetables. The NutriBullet will also take 3–4 ice cubes when added to the rest of your ingredients in a smoothie but it's not advisable to crush ice on its own. Resulting smoothies are fine and uniform in texture. The NutriBullet is very compact and convenient as you can drink straight from the blender cup that the smoothie is made in. It is easy to use, easy to clean and has a one-year guarantee. It also has a range of other containers with lids.

The Vitamix Personal Blender

This blender is at the high end of the market, but it does have a five-year warranty and the motor is quiet and built to last. The design of this model ensures ingredients are pushed towards the blades, resulting in a faster, smoother blend. It has variable speed controls and a pulse control and comes with two 0.6-litre containers and a 1.2-litre container.

OTHER EQUIPMENT

One kitchen gadget that is becoming increasingly popular is the spiraliser, which uses a razor-sharp blade to convert whole fruit and vegetables into thin ribbons and twirly strands. Courgette noodles can replace pasta, spiralised raw carrots can be added to salads and fruit spirals can be used as an interesting garnish on drinks. I recommend the Japanese-made vertical-hold Benriner Cook's Help which is available from Amazon. The blades are high quality and come in four different widths. The 1 mm blade produces super-fine strands that are great for salads. The wider 2.4 mm and 4 mm slot-in blades cut delicate taglietelle-like strips. It makes light work of even hard vegetables like beetroot and butternut squash.

Here are some other smaller items that are useful to have when making smoothies:

* Polyethylene cutting boards: many people use colour-coded boards – green for fruit, brown for vegetables
* Kitchen scales
* Sturdy bristled scrubbing brush to clean vegetables and fruit

* High-quality chopping knives, which need to be sharpened regularly
* Vegetable peeler
* Calibrated measuring jug
* Salad spinner for removing excess water from washed vegetables
* Sieve for straining thicker smoothies, if desired
* Large lidded storage jug suitable for use in the refrigerator
* Glass storage bowls with plastic lids
* Zipped plastic bags for storing washed and dried vegetables.

Using and cleaning the blender

Different blenders are operated differently so it's worth following the specific instructions for your blender and getting to know what it is capable of. However, here are a few general guidelines:

* Cut up larger fruit and vegetables.
* Put all your ingredients in the blender starting with leafy greens, then fruit, then any extra ingredients like nuts and seeds and finally liquid.
* Do not let the ingredients go higher than the max line or marker line.

Most blenders are easy to clean – just wash the removable parts by hand or, if dishwasher-safe, load in the dishwasher. If the power base gets dirty, unplug it and wipe it down with a damp cloth.

Choosing ingredients

Support your local economy and environment by finding a local fruit and vegetable farm.

I do not believe that organic foods are necessarily safer or more nutritious than inorganic. However, it is best to buy unwaxed apples and cucumbers. Cucumbers can be washed with a little soap and rinsed well and the peel left on, although it can be quite bitter.

Buy produce in bulk where appropriate. For example, you could buy freshly dug carrots by the sackload, which you can then wash and store in a cool dark place until needed. (A second refrigerator in a garage would also be very useful for storage.)

INCLUDING NUTS AND SEEDS

One of the benefits of using a blender is that you can include nuts and seeds in your drinks. Used in moderate amounts in your smoothies, nuts and seeds are nutritionally valuable foods; they contain no cholesterol, but do contain significant amounts of healthy fats, and minerals, including calcium, phosphorus, iron, zinc and magnesium. Most seeds and nuts also contain significant amounts of vitamins such as thiamine, riboflavin, niacin, folate and vitamin E. In order to reduce the phytic acid that is the protective layer that surrounds all grains, pseudo-cereals, nuts and legumes, it is recommended that they are soaked in order to activate them to start germination and reduce the phytic acid, which is an anti-nutrient that irritates the gut lining and prevents the absorption of certain minerals, especially iron, calcium and zinc into the body. This soaking will, therefore, make the nutrients more available and easier to digest. So soak the nuts or seeds overnight then rinse, drain and add the wet, softened nuts or seeds to your smoothies.

Home-made nut milks

Some recipes include almond milk as a healthy way of adding liquid to your blend. Rather than buy these in the shops, you can make your own to add to your smoothies or as a refreshing drink by itself. The following basic recipe is for making nut milks using cashews, almonds, Brazil nuts or hazelnuts. They can be sweetened with a few dates, raisins or honey in the blend, and a few seeds from a vanilla pod, or a pinch of ground Himalayan salt.

SERVES **1–2**

Ingredients
* 100 g/3½ oz blanched almonds, raw cashew nuts, Brazil nuts or hazelnuts
* 400 ml/14 fl oz water or coconut water

Soak the nuts in the water overnight. Then blend in the blender until smooth. Strain through a muslin cloth, squeezing out all the liquid, then discard the pulp. Rinse out the blender and add the strained nut milk and the sweetening agents of your choice, and blend until smooth. Refrigerate in a sealed container immediately and serve iced.

INCLUDING SEAWEED

Seaweed, also known as sea vegetables, is one of the most valuable food supplements to be found and contains 12 key minerals, in particular organic iodine. This is needed by the thyroid gland to manufacture the hormone thyroxin, which aids digestion. Iodine is also needed for brain functioning, and it kills harmful bacteria in the bloodstream. Iodine deficiency contributes to enlarged adenoids, fatigue, colds and infections.

Another important benefit of taking seaweed supplements is that the carbohydrates found in them do not elevate blood sugar levels so are suitable for people with blood sugar problems.

You can buy seaweed supplements in most health food stores under the names of seaweed, sea lettuce, kelp or dulse. Fresh or dried uncooked and unprocessed seaweed are the most beneficial and are usually supplied as powder or granules which can be sprinkled on any vegetable cocktail combinations.

SHOPPING LIST

Fruit	Mango
Apricots	Nectarine
Bananas	Orange
Black cherries	Papaya (pawpaw)
Blackcurrants	Peach
Blood orange	Pear
Blueberries or blackberries	Pink grapefruit
Cantaloupe melon	Pineapple
Dates	Raspberries
Eating (dessert) apple	Strawberries
Frozen summer fruit berry mix	Watermelon
Grapefruit	
Golden Delicious apple	**Vegetables**
Grapes (red)	Avocado
Green (tart) apple	Beetroot (red beet)
Honeydew melon	Broccoli
Kiwi	Carrots
Lemon	Cauliflower
Lime	Celery

	Extras
Courgette (zucchini)	Almond milk (unsweetened)
Cucumber	Almonds (unsalted, flaked or
Fennel bulb	whole)
Green cabbage	Apple cider vinegar
Green (bell) pepper	Coconut milk or coconut water
Jerusalem artichoke	Flaxseeds
or sweet potato	Honey
Parsnip	Ice
Potato	Japanese barley miso paste
Red (bell) pepper	Maca powder
Tomato or cherry	Maple syrup
tomatoes	Milk
Spinach or baby spinach	Oat bran
Watercress	Olive oil
	Peanut butter
Herbs and spices	Porridge oats or Mornflake
Basil, fresh	superfast oats
Cinnamon	Stevia powder
Cloves	Pumpkin or sunflower seeds
Curry powder	Sesame seeds
Garlic	Slimline ginger ale
Mint, fresh	Sugar
Nutmeg	Wheatgerm
Parsley, fresh	Wheatgrass
Root ginger	Yoghurt and Greek-style yoghurt
Turmeric, ground	

Preparing ingredients

✸ Wash all fruits and vegetables thoroughly as soon as possible after purchase. Use a vegetable scrubbing brush, if necessary.

✸ Scrub carrots rather than peeling them so that you receive the maximum nutrition from the whole vegetable.

✸ The peel, seeds and stems of some fruit and vegetables can be included in your smoothie to obtain optimum nutrition. Oranges and grapefruits, however, should be peeled but blended with as much of the white pith as possible. (The charts on pages 81–101 give more specific guidelines on the preparation of each fruit and vegetable.)

✳ Use a salad spinner to remove excess water from green vegetables.

✳ Store washed and dried prepared produce in a refrigerator or in a cool dark place in sealed plastic bags ready for use.

✳ When preparing vegetables and fruit for your smoothies, slice or dice them immediately before they are to be blended and drunk, for vitamin C losses are high on exposure to air.

Tips on consuming smoothies

✳ It is a good idea to combine fruit and vegetables in your smoothies as this helps to dilute the carb content and lowers the GI of the juice so that the impact on your blood sugar levels is less. Because it is less sweet you will be less inclined to drink too much and will take longer to drink it. (The GI is the glycemic Index which is a measurement carried out on carbohydrate-containing foods and their impact on our blood sugar.)

WHAT ABOUT THE PIPS?

In a letter to me, Peter Bazalgette says that 'there is no danger from pips pressed into apple juice. There is only a minute amount of cyanide, and it is soon dissipated into the juice. Only if someone made quantities of paste exclusively from pips could a problem arise.' (Some people, however, prefer to discard apple pips before blending as they tend to turn the smoothie slightly brown.)

✳ Many people are put off by the taste and colour of green smoothies (i.e. spinach, parsley, lettuce, Brussels sprouts, cabbage and kale). But if you include fruit or carrots with the greens it dulls the earthy taste and is much more palatable.

✳ Melons do not taste good combined with vegetables, apart from watermelons.

✳ The FODMAP (Fermentable Oligo-Di-Monosaccharides and Polyols) content of vegetables such as cabbage, kale and cauliflower can cause bloating, gas and discomfort for some people. FODMAPs are short chain carbohydrates that are poorly absorbed in the small intestine. Foods low in FODMAPs are recommended for those with IBS.

✳ Never drink more than 30–45 ml/75 g/2–3 oz of green vegetable smoothies at a time. Dilute to taste with apple or carrots.

✳ It is best to chew vegetable-based smoothies – swirl it around in your mouth until it feels warm and tastes sweet which aids absorption into your system.

✳ Try and build up to two 250 ml/8 fl oz/1 cup quantities of vegetable smoothies a day.

✳ You should always dilute vegetable and fruit juices for children with water as the neat juices are too potent for young digestive systems. Teenagers should restrict themselves to one or two 150 ml /¼ pt /²/₃ cup glasses of raw juices a day.

✳ If you are diabetic or have any other medical condition, consult your doctor before embarking on a smoothie programme. Although small quantities of unsweetened fruit juices (less than 300 ml) can be included in a diabetic diet, it must be counted as part of the carbohydrate allowance. Juice provides a lot of carbohydrates in a small portion: usually about 125 ml/4 oz or less of juice contains 15 grams of carbohydrate (one fruit portion). A combination of vegetables and fruit in your smoothies is better as the carb content will be lower. A full-on smoothie fast is definitely not suitable for a diabetic. See diabetes.co.uk for more information.

✳ Avocados with their stones removed can be blended with fruit juice smoothies or with tomato and cucumbers for green smoothies. Because the flesh of the avocado browns quickly, a little lemon or lime juice can be added.

✳ Cucumbers, courgettes and watermelons have a high water content which makes them ideal for mixing with other fruits and vegetables in smoothies, instead of apples.

✳ If you need to store your smoothie for a little while, place an ice cube in a thermos flask and fill the flask to the very top with fresh juice in the morning so that it will be ready for your lunchtime snack or a picnic. It can also be stored in the refrigerator for no more than 24 hours.

Adapting the recipes

Once you have learned how to work your blender, the fun can begin. There are plenty of recipes scattered throughout this book but you can create your own combinations of fruit and vegetable smoothies if you want to. Experiment and devise your own drinks with what you have available, and don't forget that you can give them an individual touch by adding certain herbs, such as basil, coriander, marjoram, mint and oregano, or freshly ground spices, such as allspice, cinnamon, ginger, nutmeg and liquorice root sticks. Or perhaps you might like to add the slightly salty taste of seaweed flakes. When it comes to making smoothies in the blender there are an infinite number of possibilities.

There are plenty of dairy and dairy substitutes to choose from to add liquid to your blender. For example: milk, unsweetened almond milk, coconut milk, coconut water, oat milk, rice milk, soya milk, rooibos and herbal teas. Adding yoghurt gives a creamy texture and thickens the smoothie, and is an excellent source of calcium. Greek-style yoghurt with zero per cent fat is particularly good. The soya bean curd, tofu, has a mild creamy flavour, and is said to be a good source of non-animal protein.

Fine dining and lingering over coffee and liqueurs may be a thing of the past, but you can produce delicious alcoholic sorbets and mousses in your blender in a trice; try Eton Mess with Crème de Fraise/Crème de Framboise or a refreshing Chartreuse Sorbet. For an after-dinner cocktail that aids digestion, Crème de Menthe Frappé can easily be created in a good-quality blender as it breaks up the ice very quickly.

2. Smoothies for improved health

'In future man will use the sunshine elements of plants to regenerate and heal the human body'

George Crile MD

A healthy balanced diet

A diet comprising solely of fruit and vegetable smoothies is not advocated. It is important to eat a balanced wholefood diet, and this should include daily fibre from fresh whole fruit and vegetables as well as pasta, rice, wholegrain cereals, wholemeal bread, nuts, seeds, lentils and beans.

Eating patterns have changed and eating three meals a day at home is now a thing of the past. Home-cooked meals today are largely quick and easy and often made with highly processed food items. Much depends on your budget and how much time you want to spend in the kitchen. Colour, texture and flavour all help to make food and drink enjoyable, and there is an enormous range of all three in juiced fruit and vegetable drinks.

Meals should fit in with our lifestyles: there are no hard and fast rules for individuals as to when to eat or even how much to eat, but eating at regular intervals of 5–6 hours, with no in-between snacks, is recommended. However, this does exclude diabetics, who may require snacks at certain times of the day to boost their blood sugar levels, and children and the elderly, who may not be able to consume large quantities at one meal and need snacks to boost their calorie and nutrient intake. In these cases, the vegetable drinks taken mid- or late afternoon will be an excellent pick-me-up.

Rather than relying on workplace canteens or food from shops, cafés, sandwich bars and pubs, which are often high in fat and low in fibre, working people can take in their own lunches – an effective way in controlling what you eat at midday. If you have a refrigerator or microwave at work, you can increase the range of options from prepared sandwiches to include salads and home-made soups and juiced drinks in a thermos flask. A home freezer provides an excellent opportunity to cook extra quantities of foods as standbys for busy working people.

Nutritionists have changed the traditional food wheel and now recommend a diet high in grains, fruits and vegetables, and low amounts of milk, yoghurt, cheese, meats, nuts, fats and sweets.

MEDITERRANEAN DIET

One of the most successful and disease-reducing diets in the world today is the Mediterranean diet. It consists of olive oil, pasta, unrefined cereals, potatoes, rice, legumes, fish, freshly dressed salads and cooked vegetables, large quantities of fresh fruit and vegetables, and garlic, which is now said to inhibit cancer growth. There is a moderate consumption of dairy products (mainly as cheese and yoghurt), and low consumption of lean meats. Freshly juiced fruits and vegetables can be very much a part of this healthy Mediterranean diet.

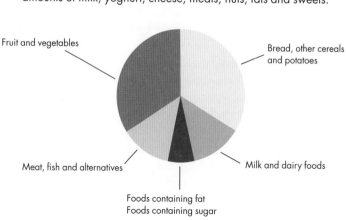

Fruit and vegetables

Bread, other cereals and potatoes

Meat, fish and alternatives

Milk and dairy foods

Foods containing fat
Foods containing sugar

JETHRO KLOSS

The correct food was prescribed by the American nutritionist Jethro Kloss, author of *Back to Eden*, the classic guide to herbal medicine and natural foods which was published in 1939 and updated and expanded in 1994. For years Kloss had successfully treated cancer patients and his book cites many cases. When asked, as he was many times, what his cancer cure was, he replied: 'Correct food, herbs, water, fresh air, massage, sunshine, exercise and rest.'

How to detox and cleanse

Consuming only smoothies over a one-, two- or three-day period is one of the ways to eliminate harmful toxins and accumulated wastes in your body that can build up because of stress or poor nutrition. A longer period of fasting is not advocated because you are likely to succumb to the need to catch up on lost food supply and consequently you can soon return to your original weight or may increase it. Those suffering from serious conditions such as diabetes or kidney disease or those undergoing chemotherapy should never attempt fasting. Elderly people should always seek medical advice before following a fasting programme. Fasting on water alone can also be dangerous and should not be attempted. It is important to make sure you drink at least 2.0–3.5 litres/4–6 pts/8–14 cups of liquid each day because of the dangers of dehydration.

When fasting, substitute for each meal one or two 250 ml/8 fl oz/1 cup quantities of vegetable or fruit smoothies, which can be diluted with mineral water. You can also make up the liquid quantity during the day with lemon and water sweetened with a little honey.

The main purpose of fasting on raw foods is to restore the body to a healthy state. The Swiss rohsaft kur (raw juice cure) is used worldwide by leading health spas, with the knowledge that it can reduce high blood pressure, and high cholesterol and uric acid levels in your bloodstream. Pounds can be shed in the process, and the skin clears and tightens. Nails become healthier and stronger, hair develops a shine and the eyes brighten. The digestive organs benefit from the rest, and the patient feels more mentally alert and active.

BODY BRUSHING

Almost a third of the body's waste products are eliminated through the skin. The health specialist Leslie Kenton recommends spending five minutes a day dry-brushing our bodies with a long-handled natural bristle brush or a rough hemp glove as an important measure to rid our bodies of harmful toxins and encourage better lymphatic circulation. With the exception of your face, brush the entire body with the dry brush or glove. For maximum benefit, take a warm shower afterwards, then switch to a 30-second cold only shower. Dry yourself and keep warm. This is an excellent method for cellulite-prone women to rid themselves of harmful toxins, though a radical change in diet and lots of exercise are also needed.

It is important to keep your fast days free and only do things that require a limited amount of energy and effort. Read a good book. If you feel the need to sleep then do so. In general, try to relax and if possible include plenty of fresh air during the day.

When breaking the fast, return to solid food gradually and then, when your body and stomach has adjusted to this new regime, return to your normal diet.

Good colon health

We spend a fortune on grooming and cleansing and looking after our external bodies and spare very little thought about the cleansing of the colon. Good colon health is vital to our everyday well-being. Although some people manage to go without passing a stool for several days, it is best for your body to have a bowel movement at least once a day, so that toxins are not collecting for too long. It is said that it takes 8–12 hours for food to be fully digested, and for all the nutrients to be absorbed, and for the waste to be eliminated. The late Dr Norman Walker stated that colon neglect is the cause of many deaths. He described the colon as 'the body's sewer' and constipation as 'our bodies' greatest enemy'.

The natural way to remedy constipation is to increase the amount of fibre in the diet, increase your water intake and take regular exercise. A doctor should be consulted if constipation persists or if a patient recognises a significant change in bowel patterns.

Adjusting to your new diet

It is important to begin slowly when introducing smoothies to your diet. The smoothie programme can be increased when your stomach and digestive system have adjusted to the new regime.

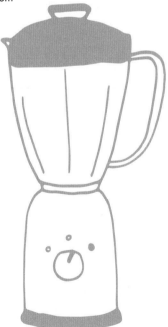

An abrupt change from a bad diet to a therapeutic diet with blended raw fruit and vegetables will definitely not agree with the digestion of most people initially. You may experience wind disturbance, bloating and sometimes diarrhoea, but rest assured that these reactions are the natural part of the detoxification process that the body has to make on its road back to health. In time, these problems will subside and, with perseverance, you will see signs of the responsive conditions taking effect.

Recipes for good health

CLEANSE AND DETOX

The smoothies in this section are a great way to start your programme as they are excellent for cleansing the liver and kidneys and flushing out any toxins as well as building blood, strengthening muscles and aiding circulation.

Body Detox V

Health benefits: This is the drink to cleanse the system. Cucumbers are a natural diuretic and beetroot (red beet) is a powerful cleanser and builder of the blood. If you include 5–7.5 cm/2–3 in of the purple stalks of the beetroot in the blender, this will give you a valuable amount of vitamin K.

Taste test: ✴ ✴ ✴
Fresh and clean; if it seems bitter add some apple cider vinegar.

SERVES **1**

Ingredients
- ✴ 1 medium carrot
- ✴ ½ cucumber
- ✴ 1 apple
- ✴ ¼ beetroot (red beet), unpeeled
- ✴ 1 tsp apple cider vinegar (optional)
- ✴ 120 ml/½ cup mineral water, or 2 ice cubes

Wash the carrot and cut it into 5–7.5 cm/2–3 in pieces. Peel the cucumber, if waxed, and cut into quarters and then into strips. Core the apple and cut into narrow wedges and the beetroot (red beet) into wedges. Process all the vegetables, the apple and the mineral water or ice cubes in the blender in short bursts, or 25 seconds at a time until smooth.

If the mixture is too thick for your liking, thin it down with more liquid or ice. Store the leftover beetroot (red beet) in a glass storage container in your refrigerator.

My verdict: ☐ ☐ ☐ ☐ ☐

BEETROOT JUICE

New research shows that having beetroot juice enhances the muscles' ability to utilise oxygen, which enhances sport performance. A small shot of 100 ml of juice is enough to give the effect. Andrew Jones, a UK professor in sports medicine, is doing this research. He has been nicknamed Andy Beetroot.

Citrus Sensation F

Health benefits: Lime and lemons are a good source of vitamin C which helps promote healthy teeth, bones and gums as well as being a good body cleanser, eliminating toxins.

Taste test: ✳ ✳ ✳ ✳ ✳
A luscious lemon-sherbet flavour; one of the most refreshing drinks you'll ever taste!

SERVES **1**

Ingredients
✳ 2 apples
✳ ¼ lime or lemon, without skin
✳ Crushed ice or mineral water

Core the apple and cut into wedges and slice the lemon or lime and remove the skin. Process the fruit in short bursts in the blender, then serve over crushed ice.

My verdict: ☐ ☐ ☐ ☐ ☐

Cucumber Cleanser V

Health benefits: This is another cleansing tonic. Dr Norman Walker, an American expert on juicing, recommended this combination for removing the uric acid of arthritis. Parsley has an astonishing amount of minerals and cumin is referred to by Pliny as the best appetiser of all the condiments. It is also said to aid digestion. After grinding, cumin powder will lose its flavour rapidly.

Taste test: ✳ ✳ ✳
Clean, sharp and peppery; the earthy flavour takes a bit of getting used to.

SERVES **1**

Ingredients
* ¼ beetroot (red beet), unpeeled
* 2 sprigs of parsley
* ½ cucumber
* 1 carrot
* 1 tsp freshly ground cumin seeds
* 1 tsp apple cider vinegar (optional)

Blend all the ingredients together in the blender.

My verdict: ☐ ☐ ☐ ☐ ☐

Strawberry Fayre F

Health benefits: Strawberries are a very good source of vitamin C and a natural sugar that cleanses the system. They are good for strengthening the blood as they are high in iron, potassium and iodine.

Taste test: ✳ ✳ ✳ ✳ ✳
Thick, creamy and perfectly scrumptious!

SERVES **1**

Ingredients
* 2 Golden Delicious or other eating (dessert) apples
* 8 strawberries
* 2 ice cubes, or crushed ice

Core the apples and cut into wedges. Hull the strawberries and process both fruits and the ice cubes through the blender, or serve over crushed ice, or over vanilla ice cream as a dessert.

My verdict: ☐ ☐ ☐ ☐ ☐

Peter Rabbit's Delight V/F

Health benefits: If Peter Rabbit had followed this recipe, he might have avoided being caught by Mr McGregor! Cabbages have ample amounts of beta-carotene, and they are loaded with other vitamins and minerals. They are tissue builders and remove toxins from the body and help digestion. The seeds add extra nutrition and a fibre boost to your drink.

Taste test: ✹ ✹ ✹
Slightly bitter but the sweet apple juice improves the taste.

SERVES **2**

Ingredients
- ✹ 1 large carrot
- ✹ 1 sweet eating (dessert) apple
- ✹ ¼ small green cabbage or a handful of kale
- ✹ ¼ cup/4 tbsp sunflower seeds, or pumpkin seeds
- ✹ 1 cup/250 ml mineral water
- ✹ 2 small ice cubes

Wash the carrot and use 5–7.5 cm/2–3 in of the green stalks and cut into pieces. Core the apple and cut into pieces, and process all the ingredients in the blender, placing the seeds on top of the blend.

My verdict: ☐ ☐ ☐ ☐ ☐

Orange Mint Marvel F

Health benefits: Blood oranges contain three times the vitamin C and carotene of an ordinary orange. Blood oranges are only available in the UK during the first three months of the year. (Pink grapefruits are also loaded with vitamin C and carotene but are available all the year round in the large supermarkets.) Vitamin C is an antioxidant that can aid in repairing tissue and healing wounds and can protect the body from the effects of free radicals, which lead to many degenerative diseases and premature ageing of skin. They also contain vitamin A, essential for the immune system and for healthy bones, teeth, skin and eyes. The mint is mainly for flavour but also aids digestion.

Taste test: ✹ ✹ ✹ ✹ ✹

The added mint gives this delicious classic combination a delightful twist.

SERVES **1**

Ingredients
* 1 eating apple
* 2 blood oranges
* A few mint leaves
* A sprig of mint to garnish

Core the apple and cut into narrow wedges. Peel the oranges, leaving as much of the white pith as possible, then cut and break them into segments. Process the fruit in the blender with a few mint leaves. Serve over crushed ice.

My verdict: ☐ ☐ ☐ ☐ ☐

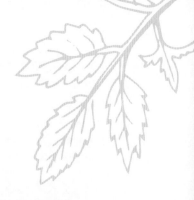

Muscle Tonic V/F

Health benefits: This could also be named Popeye's Favourite! Spinach and maca powder are both iron-rich. Iron forms part of haemoglobin, the pigment that transports oxygen from the lungs to the muscles. It is also essential for maintaining high energy levels, and it helps keep your immune system strong. Vitamin C helps with the absorption of iron and so I've included goji berries in this recipes which contain 500 times the vitamin C content per weight of oranges. Goji berries also contain up to 21 trace minerals, vitamin E, calcium and potassium. Parsley is rich in vitamin K, essential for building strong bones and preventing heart disease.

Taste test: ✴ ✴ ✴ ✴
Don't be put off by the colour of this one. It is surprisingly sweet and refreshing.

SERVES **2**

Ingredients
* 1 large carrot
* 1 apple
* 10 spinach leaves
* 4 sprigs of parsley
* 1 tbsp goji berries, pre-soaked

* 1 tsp maca powder
* 1 cup/250 ml coconut water or mineral water
* 2 ice cubes

Trim the carrots and use 5–7.5 cm/2–3 in of the green stalks, and cut into 5–7.5 cm/2–3 in pieces. Core the apple and cut into wedges. Process all the ingredients through the blender and serve in two tall glasses. Garnish with a sprig of parsley.

My verdict: ☐☐☐☐☐

Mr McGregor's Feast V

Health benefits: After a hard day in his vegetable and fruit garden Mr McGregor could have sat back in his garden and enjoyed a smoothie of the fruits of his labour. Spinach juice has a very important role to play in building the blood and revitalising the constitution, but in juicing it should only be used in moderation, once or twice a week. Kale, Swiss chard or other leafy spring greens can be a substitute. Pumpkin seeds provide further iron and healthy fats while peppers, tomatoes and celery all cleanse the body in various ways.

Taste test: ✹ ✹ ✹
Savoury and nutty.

SERVES **2**

Ingredients
* A handful of spinach
* 1 celery stalk
* 1 carrot chopped
* 2 tomatoes
* ½ green or red (bell) pepper
* 1½ tbsp soaked pumpkin or sunflower seeds
* Apple juice or almond milk
  to the max line

Place the spinach in the blender cup and add the rest of the ingredients placing the seeds on top, and fill up with the apple juice or almond milk. Blend well until smooth and thick.

My verdict: ☐☐☐☐☐

HEALTHY HEART

The British Heart Foundation recommends a healthy diet to help reduce your risk of developing coronary heart disease, diabetes and high blood pressure. They advocate at least five portions of fruit and vegetables a day as part of a well-balanced diet. In Canada and the USA they are advocating even higher intakes from seven to nine servings. This can be a lot easier to achieve if you consume these as juices or smoothies. The following recipes all contribute to a healthy heart.

Blackcurrant Booster F

Health benefits: Blackcurrants are especially rich in vitamin C, which health experts now say is vital in the prevention of cancer and heart disease. Apples too are good for the heart as they lower your cholesterol. You can substitute blackberries for the blackcurrants in this recipe, if you wish, and garnish with a few raspberries and raspberry leaves.

Taste test:
Rich in flavour and colour; lively, sharp and utterly delectable.

SERVES **2**

Ingredients
* 175 g/6 oz blackcurrants
* 5 sweet eating (dessert) apples
* 6 mint leaves, chopped
* 20 ml/4 tsp clear honey
* 2 blackcurrant sprigs dipped in caster (superfine) sugar, to garnish

Wash and drain the blackcurrants and top and tail them. Cut the apples into wedges and blend with the blackcurrants and mint. Add honey to taste. Pour into two tall glasses and garnish each with a sprig of blackcurrants.

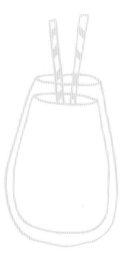

My verdict: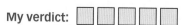

Hearty Oats and Berries **F**

Health benefits: Oats are bursting with natural goodness, and are 100 per cent wholegrain. They are high in fibre and oat beta glucans, which have been shown to help to actively lower cholesterol, and may reduce the risk of coronary heart disease. The berries and yoghurt in this smoothie also promote a healthy heart. Coconut water is very high in potassium and is now available in most supermarkets.

Taste test: ✳ ✳ ✳ ✳
Refreshing, tangy and oaty; a perfect breakfast drink.

SERVES **2**

Ingredients
- ✳ 3 tbsp porridge oats or Mornflake superfast oats
- ✳ ½ x 500 g pack frozen summer fruit berry mix
- ✳ 150 g Greek-style yoghurt with honey
- ✳ 100 ml apple juice (using home juicer) or coconut water

Toast the oats in a small non-stick frying pan for five minutes until golden. Place the smoothie berry mix straight from the freezer into the blender, with the yoghurt, apple juice or coconut water and 2½ tbsp of the oats and whizz until smooth and thick. Pour into two glasses and serve with the remaining toasted oats over the top.

My verdict: ☐ ☐ ☐ ☐ ☐

Purple Power **V/F**

Health benefits: Here is another recipe containing blackcurrants that are rich in vitamin C, a protection against cancer and heart disease. Beetroot (red beet) is rich in nitrates which our body converts into nitrate oxide, a chemical thought to lower blood pressure. It contains many other necessary vitamins and micronutrients that support and purify our body cells. Coconut milk contains magnesium which aids in circulation and keeps muscles relaxed – important in the prevention of heart attacks.

Taste test: ✳ ✳ ✳ ✳

Full-flavoured fruitiness that overrides the earthiness of the beetroot.

SERVES **1**

Ingredients
* ❋ 115 g beetroot (red beet), peeled and cut into chunks
* ❋ 130 g frozen or fresh blackcurrants
* ❋ 300 ml coconut milk

Cut the beetroot (red beet) into chunks and blend with the rest of the ingredients until smooth.

My verdict: ☐ ☐ ☐ ☐ ☐

Cardio Kiwi **F**

Health benefits: Kiwis are packed with vitamins and minerals. They contain potassium and almost twice as much vitamin C as oranges. Potassium and vitamin C both help to keep blood pressure at a normal level. Kiwis also contain a small amount of vitamin E: a potent antioxidant said to help lower cholesterol and boost immunity.

Taste test: ❋ ❋ ❋ ❋ ❋
The sweetness of the apples mingles with the tartness of the kiwi in this delicious, creamy concoction.

SERVES **1**

Ingredients
* ❋ 2 Golden Delicious apples
* ❋ 3 kiwi fruit, peeled
* ❋ Crushed ice

Core the apples and cut into narrow wedges, and the peeled kiwis into halves. Process the fruit in the blender. Serve over crushed ice.

My verdict: ☐ ☐ ☐ ☐ ☐

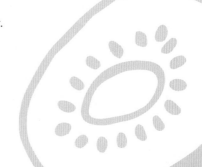

Super Commuter ▮F▮

Health benefits: This smoothie has the busy office commuter in mind – a breakfast you can grab and go that will last you three to four days (see below). Plus papaya, banana, hemp seeds, sunflower seeds and maca powder are all known for being beneficial in keeping your heart healthy. Maca also has the added benefits of increasing energy and stamina and improving your mood. It is also helpful for women with menopausal problems. That should set you up for the day!

Taste test: ✹ ✹ ✹ ✹ ✹
Delicious banana and butterscotch combo.

This is a condensed refrigerated recipe, enough for 3–4 days. It can be diluted to the water level line in the blenders for each day's serving. A ready-mixed portion can be stored in a flask overnight for busy office commuter travellers!

Ingredients
- ✹ 3 tsp maca powder
- ✹ 2 tbsp hemp seeds or organic linseeds
- ✹ 2 tbsp sunflower seeds
- ✹ A large papaya (pawpaw), peeled and deseeded, cut into cubes
- ✹ 1 frozen or freshly peeled banana
- ✹ 2 tbsp unsweetened Greek-style yogurt

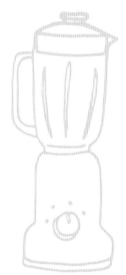

Mix all the above ingredients in the blender for 25 or 30 seconds until well blended.

Add any of the following liquids to the water line level in the blender for each serving: roasted almond milk, coconut milk, full cream milk or semi-skimmed milk for a creamier taste or coconut water or spring water plus 4–5 ice cubes.

My verdict: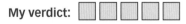

HEALTHY LUNGS

Fruit and vegetables are a great source of vitamins and minerals that can help prevent chest infections or help you fight them off more quickly. Those people with lung conditions can feel too breathless to eat very much and chewing can be difficult. Drinking juices and smoothies will give you the vitamins and minerals you need with less effort as you consume them.

Lusty Lungs V

Health benefits: Watercress is a good source of calcium and magnesium. It is good for cleansing the lungs of toxins, and respiratory infections are said to benefit from doses of watercress juice. The carotenoids in the carrots and the watercress help prevent lung cancer and potatoes contain vitamin B6, good for overall lung health.

Taste test: ✳ ✳ ✳ ✳ ✳

Beautifully sweet with a hint of pepperiness. Surprisingly, the potato doesn't dominate.

SERVES **1–2**

Ingredients
✳ 1 apple
✳ 4 sprigs watercress
✳ ¼ potato, unpeeled
✳ 2 medium carrots
✳ 4 sprigs parsley
✳ 1 cup/250 ml mineral water
✳ 2 ice cubes

Core the apple and cut into wedges. Blend together with all the other ingredients.

My verdict: ☐ ☐ ☐ ☐ ☐

Carrot Combat V

Health benefits: Carrots are rich in vitamin A, vitamin C and lycopene, all antioxidants that affect lung health and lower the chances of developing lung disease and prostate cancer. Apples are rich in flavonoids, vitamin E and vitamin C which help the lungs function at their best. Ginger works as an expectorant to rid the sinus cavities of mucus and the lungs of phlegm. The coconut water will supply you with extra potassium, and the green carrot stalks a useful amount of vitamin K.

Taste test: ✳ ✳ ✳ ✳
A tasty sweet and spicy blend to tickle your taste buds.

SERVES **1**

Ingredients
✳ 2 carrots (including stalks)
✳ 1 apple
✳ 2.5 cm/1 in piece of root ginger
✳ 1 cup/250 ml coconut water, or mineral water
✳ 2 ice cubes

Cut the carrots and their stalks into 5–7.5cm/2–3 in pieces. Core the apple into narrow wedges. Slice the ginger root into a few pieces. Process all the ingredients through the blender.

My verdict: ☐ ☐ ☐ ☐ ☐

NATURAL BEAUTY AND HEALTHY EYES

Once you start juicing on a regular basis, you will notice a significant improvement in your skin, which will become more radiant. Your hair will look shinier, your eyes brighter and your nails stronger. The following recipes will become the staple for maintaining natural beauty and looking younger for longer.

Carrot Cocktail V/F

Health benefits: Carrots are a rich source of beta-carotene, which among other vital uses can be converted into vitamin A in the body to maintain healthy skin, hair and nails.

Taste test: ✹ ✹ ✹ ✹
Adding the apple to carrot juice makes it sweeter and much more palatable.

SERVES **1**

Ingredients
✹ 2 carrots
✹ 2 apples
✹ 1 cup/250 ml mineral water
✹ 2 ice cubes

Trim the carrots and cut them into 5–7.5 cm/2–3 in pieces. Cut the apple into wedges and process all the ingredients through the blender.

My verdict: ☐ ☐ ☐ ☐ ☐

Mango Tango F

Health benefits: Mangos are rich in beta-carotene, potassium, vitamin C and vitamin B6. They help clear clogged pores that cause acne, and add freshness to the face. Mangos are also good for the relief of constipation and indigestion.

Taste test: ✹ ✹ ✹ ✹ ✹

A thick, super-sweet and delicious juice; the level of sweetness can be toned down with tarter apples.

SERVES **1**

Ingredients
- ✳ 1 mango
- ✳ 1 apple

Pick the larger varieties of mangos for those with most juice. Halve the mango, remove the stone (pit) and slice the flesh from the skin. Cut the mango flesh into strips. Cut the apple into wedges and process both fruits in the juicer. If the mixture is too thick slacken with a little coconut water.

My verdict: ☐ ☐ ☐ ☐ ☐

Apricot Glow   F/V

Health benefits: Apricots contain silicon which promotes healthy skin and hair and melons are rich in vitamins A, and B-complex vitamins which are also vital for healthy skin. The vitamin E in the sunflower seeds combats UV rays and keeps skin youthful.

Taste test: ✳ ✳ ✳ ✳ ✳
A peaches-and-cream combination of exciting flavours.

SERVES **2**

Ingredients
- ✳ 1 carrot, diced
- ✳ ½ cantaloupe melon, peeled, seeded and chopped
- ✳ 4 apricots, pitted
- ✳ 1 tsp sunflower seeds (optional)
- ✳ 2 tsp runny honey
- ✳ A little unsweetened almond milk to the water line
- ✳ 2 ice cubes

Place all the ingredients in the blender and blend until smooth.

My verdict: ☐ ☐ ☐ ☐ ☐

Punchy Parsnip V

Health benefits: Parsnips are a good source of vitamin C, vitamin E, chlorine, phosphorous, potassium, silicon and sulphur, so they are good for the nutrition of the skin, hair and nails. Carrots and parsley not only keep your eyes bright but are also an aid to good eyesight. The spices in curry powder have health benefits such as the anti-inflammatory effect of turmeric.

Taste test: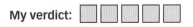
Similar to curried parsnip soup, the carrots and parsnip give this a pleasantly sweet flavour while the curry powder adds a bit of extra zing. You can increase the curry powder for a hotter drink.

SERVES **2**

Ingredients

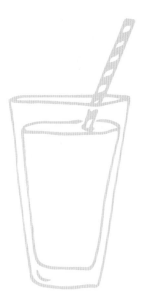

* 1 carrot
* 1 apple
* ¼ parsnip
* 4 sprigs of parsley
* ½ tsp mild curry powder
* Soya wholebean unsweetened milk to the max line
* 2 ice cubes

Cut the carrots and their green stalks into 5–7.5 cm/2–3 in pieces. Core the apple and cut into narrow wedges; cut the parsnip into strips. Process all the other ingredients through the blender.

My verdict: ☐ ☐ ☐ ☐ ☐

Eye Elixir **V**

Health benefits: When it comes to our eyes we don't just want them to look bright, we want good vision too! Carrots are full of the vitamin beta-carotene, which is renowned for improving the eyesight. Fennel contains vitamins A and C, antioxidants that can protect your eyes against certain types of eye conditions such as macular degeneration. Parsley is a powerful herb that can be used for weak eyes, cataracts and conjunctivitis.

Taste test: ✸ ✸ ✸ ✸
Light, sweet and refreshing.

SERVES **1**

Ingredients
- ✸ 2 carrots
- ✸ ¼ fennel bulb
- ✸ 4 sprigs parsley
- ✸ 1 tsp organic Japanese barley miso paste (optional)
- ✸ 1 cup/250 ml mineral water
- ✸ 1 ice cube

Cut the carrots into 5–7.5 cm /2–3 in pieces. Slice the fennel bulb using some of the leaves for extra flavour. Process both though the blender with the parsley sprigs.

NB Organic Japanese barley miso paste has a savoury yet slightly sweet taste, which enriches the flavours of soups, stews, sauces and spreads as well as in vegetable smoothies.

My verdict: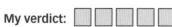

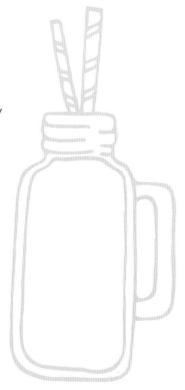

GOOD DIGESTION

As we get older, our digestive system is not as effective as it once was and can encounter more problems with indigestion, acid reflux, flatulence, diarrhoea and constipation. Here are a range of smoothies that tackle some of these issues effectively.

Apple Aniseed V/F

Health benefits: Fennel, from the same family as celery and parsley, is high in vitamins and minerals but simple to digest. It helps relieve gas and bloating quickly since it acts as an anti-spasmatic agent in the colon. It also helps relax stomach muscles and reduce any pain associated with digestion. Its juice can be mixed with beetroot (red beet), carrot or apple juice.

Taste test: ✺ ✺ ✺ ✺ ✺
A gorgeous pale green, and the wonderful taste of aniseed makes this a firm favourite.

SERVES **1**

Ingredients
- ✳ 1 small fennel bulb (approx. 100 g/4 oz)
- ✳ 2 apples
- ✳ 1 cup/250 ml natural yoghurt
- ✳ 2 tsp fennel seeds
- ✳ 1 ice cube

Core the apples and cut into wedges, and slice the fennel removing the core from each wedge. Process all the ingredients through the blender and serve.

My verdict: ☐ ☐ ☐ ☐ ☐

Hawaiian Sunrise **F**

Health benefits: This wonderful drink suggests waking up on some tropical island. Pineapples contain many minerals: manganese, calcium, chlorine, traces of iodine and iron, magnesium, phosphorus, potassium and sodium. They are rich in vitamins too, and a certain enzyme that aids digestion. Grapefruit is rich in vitamin C and in the minerals calcium, phosphorous and potassium. It is also excellent for solving problems with indigestion as it improves the flow of digestive juices.

Taste test: ✹ ✹ ✹ ✹ ✹
A tangy, tropical fruit-burst; absolutely delicious!

SERVES **1**

Ingredients
- ✹ ¼ grapefruit
- ✹ 1 pineapple round, 2.5 cm/1 in thick
- ✹ 1 eating (dessert) apple
- ✹ A small slice of lime, skin removed
- ✹ ½ cup/125 ml coconut water
- ✹ 1 tsp runny honey (optional)
- ✹ 1 ice cube

Choose fresh fruit (old fruit can be woody and dry) and if you do not use all the pineapple at once, store it in a glass container in the refrigerator, but it is better to juice and consume it as soon as possible.

Peel the grapefruit, leaving on as much white pith as possible. Cut or break the grapefruit into segments. Remove and discard the skin of the pineapple and, for optimum nutrition, cut the pineapple into 2.5 cm/1 in thick rounds and then into strips. Core the apple and cut into narrow wedges. Process all the ingredients in the blender.

NB For a potassium-enriched smoothie add a banana to the mix. If it's too thick, add some coconut milk or coconut water.

My verdict: ☐ ☐ ☐ ☐ ☐

Cherry Aid **F**

Health benefits: Cherry juice is an excellent aid to digestion and is also said to be helpful in cases of arthritis, anaemia, menstrual problems and prostate disorders. It contains beta-carotene and vitamin C and many minerals including trace elements of zinc. It is quite strong so mix with equal parts of water or apple juice.

Taste test: ✳ ✳ ✳ ✳

Deep, rich colour and wonderfully sweet and satisfying.

SERVES **1**

Ingredients
* 6 oz/170 g black cherries, stones (pits) pitted
* 1 sweet (dessert) apple
* ½ cup/150 ml unsweetened almond milk
* 1 ice cube
* A sprig of mint to garnish

Core and slice the apples and mix with the rest of the ingredients in the blender. Garnish with the sprig of mint.

My verdict: ☐ ☐ ☐ ☐ ☐

MAX BIRCHER-BENNER

Max Bircher-Benner, the Swiss physician and pioneer of nutritional science, found raw apples highly beneficial in the treatment of digestive disorders and infections. His famous clinic in Zurich, founded in 1897, still flourishes today and advocates raw juice therapy among its treatments for serious illnesses.

Ginger Digest **F**

Health benefits: Like apple, pears contain a lot of pectin, a digestive aid that helps regulate the body. Pears cleanse the body of toxins by stimulating bowel activity. With added ginger, which also helps to get things moving, this is an ideal drink if you are suffering from constipation.

Taste test: ✳ ✳ ✳ ✳ ✳
Sweet and refreshing with a zesty ginger-kick.

SERVES **1**

Ingredients
✳ 1 (dessert) apple
✳ 1 pear
✳ 2.5 cm/1 in piece of root ginger
✳ ½ cup/125 ml mineral water
✳ 1 ice cube
✳ A sprig of mint, to garnish

Core the apple and pear and cut into narrow wedges. Slice the ginger root and process all the ingredients through the blender. Garnish with the sprig of mint.

My verdict: ☐ ☐ ☐ ☐ ☐

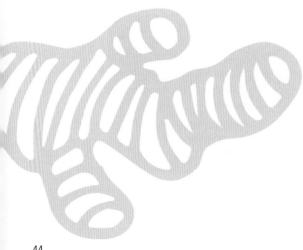

INCREASED ENERGY

Life takes a lot out of us: whether we're in a demanding job, looking after energetic children or grandchildren or are facing stressful situations, these things can lead to us feeling tired and lacking in energy. Physical exertion also takes its toll and we can suffer from muscle pain and cramps. All the recipes in this section are aimed at addressing some of these issues.

Breakfast Unblocker F

If your bowels are a bit sluggish in the mornings, this is a great way to get things moving as the oat bran and dates are both good sources of fibre. The probiotics in the yoghurt also help to regulate the digestive system and decrease gas, diarrhoea, constipation and bloating. Dates also provide you with iron and folic acid, and they add a sweetness to the drink.

Taste test: ✳ ✳ ✳ ✳ ✳
A delicious alternative to the usual breakfast fare.

SERVES **2**

Ingredients
- ✳ 2 bananas
- ✳ 1 tsp honey
- ✳ 2 tbsp oat bran
- ✳ 4 soft Deglet Nour ready-to-eat dates, pitted
- ✳ 250 ml/1 cup organic skimmed milk
- ✳ 250 ml/1 cup organic low fat yoghurt
- ✳ ¼ tsp freshly ground nutmeg, a little extra for garnish

Peel the bananas and chop the flesh. Process with the rest of the ingredients in the blender.

My verdict: ☐ ☐ ☐ ☐ ☐

Early Energiser V

Health benefits: When it's hard to get going in the morning, this is the juice to give you the boost you need. Along with the celery juice, the maca powder increases your body's resistance to external toxins and strengthens a weakened immune system. The cucumber is a good source of vitamin B needed for energy production and being 95 per cent water it is excellent at rehydrating the body.

Taste test: ✳ ✳ ✳ ✳
An appetising pale green; subtle, light and refreshing.

SERVES **1**

Ingredients
✳ ½ a cucumber
✳ 4 sticks of celery
✳ 4 sprigs of mint
✳ 1 level tsp maca powder
✳ 1 tsp apple cider vinegar (optional)

Peel and discard the skin of the cucumber if it's waxed. Blend all the ingredients together in the blender.

My verdict: ☐ ☐ ☐ ☐ ☐

IMPROVING HEALTH

Blueberry Burst F

Health benefits: Blueberries are packed with vitamins and minerals; one of these is manganese which converts carbohydrates and fats into energy. Almonds, pumpkin and sesame seeds have an anti-inflammatory effect.

Taste test: ✳ ✳ ✳ ✳
Predominantly creamy and nutty with subtle fruit flavours when using blueberries.

SERVES **2**

Ingredients
✳ 35 g raw flaked or whole unsalted almonds (skinned)
✳ 40 g raw unsalted pumpkin seeds

* 10 g raw sesame seeds
* 30 g blueberries or blackberries
* 60 ml mineral water
* 375 ml unsweetened almond milk
* 60 g honey
* 250 g ice

Place all the ingredients in the order listed above in the blender, and blend for 60 seconds until smooth and thick.

My verdict: ☐☐☐☐☐☐

Vitamin Vitality F

Health benefits: Maca powder, an ancient root from the mountains of Peru, is noted for its ability to help increase stamina, energy and sexual function. It is packed with B vitamins and a good source of iron, and it helps to restore red blood cells and aids healing and muscle pain. Apricots also give energy, stamina and endurance and avocados contain a wide variety of nutrients including potassium which helps boost energy levels.

Taste test: ✹ ✹ ✹ ✹ ✹
Sweet, nutty and creamy nectar.

MAKES **1 LITRE**

Ingredients
* 850 ml unsweetened almond milk
* 4 apricots stoned (pitted)
* 100 g apple peeled and cored
* 150 g avocado, peeled and stoned (pitted)
* 10 g fresh mint leaves
* 15 g maca powder
* Juice of ½ a lime

Place in a jug blender and blitz until smooth. Serve in glasses over ice.

My verdict: ☐☐☐☐☐☐

Green Tureen V

Health benefits: This cold soup is packed with energy-boosting vitamins and minerals. The sodium-potassium balance in celery helps alleviate muscle cramping and fatigue. The green (bell) pepper, spinach, courgette (zucchini) and cucumber are all aids to muscle problems and alleviate inflammation of conditions like arthritis. Avocados contain potassium which boosts our energy levels and the amino acids in the apple cider vinegar act as an antidote to lactic acid in the body which causes fatigue.

Taste test: ✳ ✳ ✳ ✳
You can almost taste each ingredient in this flavoursome, savoury blend similar to gazpacho soup.

SERVES **2-3**

Ingredients
* ✳ ½ cucumber, peeled (not skinned) and sliced
* ✳ 1 courgette (zucchini), pared and sliced
* ✳ 1 stick of celery, pared to remove strings
* ✳ ½ green (bell) pepper, sliced
* ✳ A small handful of baby spinach leaves
* ✳ 2 cloves of garlic
* ✳ 1 avocado
* ✳ The leaves from a sprig of mint
* ✳ The juice of ½ a lemon
* ✳ 1 tbsp extra virgin olive oil
* ✳ 200 ml iced water
* ✳ 1 tsp apple cider vinegar

Put the sliced cucumber and courgette (zucchini) in a colander and sprinkle on a heaped teaspoon of salt. Shake the colander to distribute the salt then place over a bowl. After half an hour rinse under the cold tap and pat dry with kitchen towel. Place in a blender or liquidiser with all the other ingredients and blend until smooth. If the soup is too thick, add more water. Season with salt and put in the fridge or freezer to chill the soup to icy cold. To serve: garnish with a few mint leaves, sliced green olives, and add a lump of ice and a little squiggle of olive oil to each bowl.

My verdict: ☐ ☐ ☐ ☐ ☐

APPLE CIDER VINEGAR

Apple cider vinegar should not be confused with white distilled vinegar, wine vinegar or malt vinegar, which contain acetic acid. These vinegars harm the system and destroy red blood cells which can lead to anaemia. They also interfere with digestive processes, preventing the proper absorption of foods. These vinegars are a product of fermentation of alcoholic fluids such as fermented wine and malt liquors. Acetic acid in these vinegars has been known to be a contributing factor in causing cirrhosis of the liver, duodenal and other intestinal ulcers.

Apple cider vinegar, however, is made from whole apples and not diluted. It contains malic acid that aids digestion, promotes healthy blood and combines with alkaline elements and minerals in the body, for example iron, which produces energy.

Banana Bonanza **F**

Health benefits: Bananas release energy slowly, keeping you going for longer. Peanut butter and sunflower seeds both contain vitamin E which works as an antioxidant. Peanut butter also contains magnesium which is good for building and repairing muscles and potassium for energy. Blueberries are low in calories and high in nutrients; they reduce inflammation but also aid with memory loss and are anti-ageing.

Taste test: ✹ ✹ ✹ ✹

A delicious, creamy, banana-flavoured smoothie with a hint of peanut butter.

SERVES **2**

- ✹ 1 tbsp sunflower seeds or Omega mixed seeds
- ✹ 1 banana
- ✹ ½ cup/120 ml blueberries
- ✹ 1 tbsp peanut butter
- ✹ 1 tsp honey
- ✹ ½ cup/120 ml plain yoghurt
- ✹ 1 cup/250 ml unsweetened almond milk
- ✹ 2 ice cubes

Place all the ingredients in a blender jug, and blend in short bursts until smooth.

My verdict: ☐ ☐ ☐ ☐ ☐

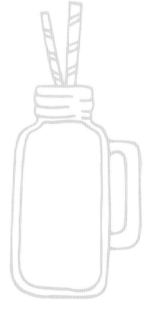

STAY CALM AND SLEEP TIGHT

Many things in life can cause us to feel anxious, stressed, run down and below par. This in turn can lead to depression and insomnia. The recipes in this section have been chosen with this in mind.

Pepper Pick-me-up V

Health benefits: Peppers, wheatgrass and cabbage are good for anxiety and stress and tomatoes are said to help with depression. The wheatgrass is loaded with chlorophyll and minerals and many nutrition counsellors use it to treat anxiety and depression because they claim it aids your body in producing its own serotonin.

Taste test: ✹ ✹ ✹
Pleasant and savoury, a bit like tomato soup; the red pepper adds extra zip.

SERVES **1**

Ingredients
- ✹ 1 red (bell) pepper
- ✹ 1 tomato
- ✹ 1 large carrot
- ✹ 40 g/1½ oz wheatgrass or ¼ sweetheart cabbage
- ✹ ½ tsp salt

Blend all the ingredients together and if required thin with a little mineral water.

My verdict: ☐ ☐ ☐ ☐ ☐

Celery Soother V

Health benefits: The organic sodium (salt) in celery is said to be good for nervous disorders and insomnia. Parsley also helps with anxiety and tomatoes contain lycopene, an antioxidant that reduces stress and can help with depression. Magnesium in sunflower seeds also helps relieve stress. The greener the stalks in the celery, the more nutritious they are. Much beta-carotene lies in the green leaves, which people often discard, and there are many vitamins and minerals in the stalks.

Taste test: ✳ ✳ ✳
Not the most appetising colour but refreshing to the palate.

SERVES **2**

Ingredients
* ✳ 4 sprigs of parsley
* ✳ A handful of green celery leaves
* ✳ 2 green celery stalks
* ✳ 2 cherry vine tomatoes
* ✳ 1½ tbsp of pre-soaked sunflower seeds
* ✳ 1 cup/250 ml soya wholebean milk or unsweetened almond milk
* ✳ 1 tsp organic apple cider vinegar
* ✳ 2 ice cubes
* ✳ 1 sprig of parsley to garnish

Process all the ingredients together and blend until smooth. Pour into two glasses and garnish with the sprig of parsley.

My verdict: ☐ ☐ ☐ ☐ ☐

Strawberry Slumber F

Health benefits: Bananas and yoghurt are high in tryptophan which promotes sleep. Also the calcium in yoghurt and milk help to relax you but if you choose to use almond milk instead, you will still reap the benefits as it contains magnesium, which has the same effect. Vitamin B6 found in strawberries is known for helping you to fall asleep.

Taste test: ✳ ✳ ✳ ✳ ✳
Pretty pink and perfectly delectable!

SERVES **2**

Ingredients
* ✳ 1 peeled and chopped banana

* 300 g/10½ oz strawberries
* 125 ml/4¼ fl oz semi-skimmed milk or unsweetened almond milk
* 150 ml/5 fl oz vanilla yoghurt
* 125 ml/4¼ fl oz apple juice or mineral water
* 6 ice cubes

Place all the ingredients in the blender and blend until smooth.

My verdict: ☐ ☐ ☐ ☐ ☐

Bedtime Broccoli V

Health benefits: Broccoli is a good all-rounder and has many health benefits as it is exceedingly high in beta-carotene, vitamins C, E and B1, is high in calcium, potassium and magnesium and has traces of selenium. The vitamin C and magnesium in broccoli (which is also present in the parsley and carrots in this recipe) helps with sleeping problems. Broccoli is also said to be good for anxiety.

Taste test: ✳ ✳ ✳ ✳
The earthy flavour of the broccoli is offset by the sweetness of the carrots and apple.

SERVES **1–2**

Ingredients
* 2 carrots
* 3–4 broccoli florets with stems
* ½ apple
* 4 sprigs of parsley
* ½ cup/140 ml soya bean milk
* 1 ice cube

Cut the carrots into 5–7.5 cm/2–3 in pieces. Slice the broccoli florets into strips. Cut the apple into narrow wedges. Process the vegetables and apple, parsley and soya bean milk through the blender with the ice cube.

My verdict: ☐ ☐ ☐ ☐ ☐

Pink Nightcap `F`

Grapefruit are a very high source of vitamin C, calcium, phosphorous and potassium. Pink grapefruit are sweeter than white and contain 49 times more beta-carotene. They also contain lycopene which can help if you suffer from sleeplessness.

Taste test: ✹ ✹ ✹ ✹
Mouth-wateringly good and full of flavour.

SERVES **1–2**

Ingredients
- ✹ 1 pink grapefruit
- ✹ ½ sweet eating (dessert) apple
- ✹ 1 ice cube

Peel the grapefruit, leaving on as much white pith as possible, and cut or break the grapefruit into segments and remove the pips (pits). Core the apple and cut into wedges, and blend with the grapefruit and ice until smooth.

My verdict: ☐ ☐ ☐ ☐ ☐

ZESTY SEX

Of course, your sex life won't just be down to what smoothies you consume! However, the recipes in this section are known to get you in the mood and improve performance.

Venus Awakened `F`

Health benefits: Good circulation is thought to be crucial for sexual functioning in both men and women, and strawberries and raspberries are rich in antioxidants that benefit your heart and arteries. What's more, they're rich in vitamin C, which along with antioxidants has been linked to higher sperm counts in men. No wonder the perfumed strawberry is the symbol of Venus, Roman goddess of love!

Taste test: ✹ ✹ ✹ ✹
If you like them tart, this is the one for you! If not, add a little honey.

SERVES **1**

Ingredients
- ✹ 12 strawberries
- ✹ 1 nectarine
- ✹ 50 g/2 oz raspberries
- ✹ 1 ice cube

Hull the strawberries. Halve the nectarine and remove the stone (pit). Blend all the fruit together with the ice cube. Strain the blend through a sieve and serve.

My verdict: ☐ ☐ ☐ ☐ ☐

Sex Enhancer F

Health benefits: Several vegetables are known to be libido-enhancers, such as celery, carrots, asparagus and fennel. Celery was popular in France in the eighteenth century for its ability to increase sexual desire and improve performance. Today, scientists have found it contains pheromones, which stimulate the sex senses. Juices rich in B vitamins, vitamin E, zinc and iodine are said to give you more zest for sex.

Taste test: ✹ ✹ ✹
The sweet liquorice flavour of the fennel mingles with the slight bitterness from the celery.

SERVES **1**

Ingredients
- ✹ 4 celery sticks
- ✹ ½ sweet eating (dessert) apple
- ✹ ¼ fennel bulb

Core the apple and cut into wedges. Cut the fennel into strips and blend all the ingredients through the blender until smooth.

My verdict: ☐ ☐ ☐ ☐ ☐

RAPID REMEDIES

Whether you have a cold or flu, are recovering from a stomach upset, have over-indulged in too much alcohol or are just feeling under the weather, one of these juices should quickly aid in your recovery and put back the spring in your step.

Ginger Fizz F

Health benefits: Apart from being a terrific source of pectin, which removes toxins from the intestines, the potassium and phosphorus in apples help flush the kidneys and control digestive upsets like diarrhoea and help you to get your appetite back.

Taste test: ✹ ✹ ✹ ✹
A sweet and very palatable drink.

SERVES **1**

Ingredients
- ✹ 3 eating (dessert) apples
- ✹ Crushed ice
- ✹ Slimline ginger ale

Core the apples and cut into narrow wedges, then process the fruit in the blender until very smooth. Serve over crushed ice in a tall glass, and top up with the slimline ginger ale to taste.

My verdict: ☐ ☐ ☐ ☐ ☐

Raspberry Reviver F

Health benefits: Raspberries are recommended for those suffering from fatigue or depression and for cooling the effects of a feverish condition. This juice is very high in vitamin C and has useful amounts of many minerals.

Taste test: ✹ ✹ ✹ ✹
A little on the sour side but very refreshing.

SERVES **1**

Ingredients
* 1 apple
* 225 g/8 oz fresh raspberries
* Crushed ice

Core the apple and cut into narrow wedges and process with the raspberries in the blender. Sieve the blend and add ½ tsp stevia powder, or honey if too tart. Serve over crushed ice.

My verdict: ☐ ☐ ☐ ☐ ☐

Capital C **F**

Health benefits: This pick-me-up smoothie contains four fruits packed with vitamin C which will give you a boost when you are feeling low in energy or spirit, or if you feel a cold coming on.

Taste test: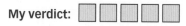

This cerise nectar is sharp and full of berry deliciousness.

SERVES **2**

Ingredients
* 150 g/5¼ oz blackcurrants or blackberries
* 150 g/5¼ oz seedless red grapes
* 2 kiwi fruit, peeled
* 1 large oranges, peeled and chopped
* 1 ice cube

Place all the ingredients in the blender. Strain through a sieve, pour into two glasses and serve immediately. This also works equally well in a juicer. Thin with a little mineral water if required.

My verdict: ☐ ☐ ☐ ☐ ☐

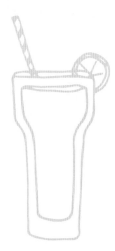

Hangover Harmony F

Health benefits: Much of the misery of a hangover is caused by dehydration, so it makes sense to flush out the alcohol from your system by drinking plenty of liquids and raise your energy levels with vitamin C fruit juices. This will also replace vitamin B1, which is depleted by alcohol.

Taste test: ✹ ✹ ✹ ✹ ✹
Clean-tasting, refreshing and hydrating.

SERVES **1**

Ingredients
✹ ¼ watermelon
✹ ¼ slice of lime
✹ 1 ice cube

Peel the watermelon and lime and cut into pieces. Blend with the ice cube.

My verdict: ☐ ☐ ☐ ☐ ☐

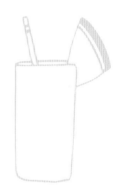

Hangover Horizon V/F

Health benefits: Vegetable juices high in vitamin C are the answer to a hangover. Carrots cleanse the liver and kidneys and rid the body of toxins and, with the celery and orange juices here, restore the vitamin C that is so depleted by alcohol.

Taste test: ✹ ✹ ✹ ✹
Cool, sweet, refreshing and thirst-quenching.

SERVES **1**

Ingredients
✹ 1 carrot
✹ 1 celery stick
✹ 1 orange
✹ A little wheatgerm (optional) for garnish
✹ 1 tsp Worcestershire sauce (optional)

Cut the carrot and celery into 5–7.5 cm/2–3 in pieces. Segment the orange, add the Worcestershire sauce and blend. Scatter the wheatgerm over the top, if wished.

My verdict: ☐☐☐☐☐

FOR DIABETICS

Diabetes is a group of metabolic disorders. Type 2 diabetes is a common health condition. It is characterised by the body's inability to manufacture or process insulin, a hormone that plays an important role in in the regulation of blood sugar levels and the energy it provides. These three tasty recipes will help those with diabetes, but can be enjoyed by all.

Firmly Rooted V

Health benefits: Jerusalem artichokes, available in the autumn, make a useful juice for diabetics as they are loaded with natural inulin (not insulin). Inulin is a type of dietary fibre, a soluble fibre, which helps to slow the rise of one's blood sugar levels. Sweet potatoes and sunflower seeds are also good for a diabetic diet. Artichokes are a very good source of potassium and this smoothie also contains vitamins B6, C, D and magnesium.

Taste test: ✳ ✳ ✳ ✳ ✳
Wonderful creamy, nutty flavour.

SERVES **2**

Ingredients
* 145 g steamed Jerusalem artichoke or sweet potato
* 250 ml unsweetened almond milk
* 30 ml maple syrup or 1 tsp stevia powder
* 3 g milled sunflower seeds
* 1 g/¼ tsp ground turmeric
* 200 g ice

You can leave the skin on artichokes and on sweet potatoes, but make sure you scrub them well if you do. Steam the artichokes for about 5 to 8 minutes (sweet potatoes for about 15 to 20 minutes) then leave to cool. Place all the ingredients in the order listed above in the blender for 25 seconds. Adjust the sweetening to your taste.

My verdict: ☐☐☐☐☐

Peppy Papaya F

Health benefits: Papaya (pawpaw) is very high in vitamins A and C. It also protects against heart disease, and kidney and liver disorders. Papaya (pawpaw) is an intermediate GI fruit but the green apples, flaxseeds and yoghurt help to slow the rise in one's blood sugar levels. Cinnamon is also very effective in doing this. Papaya (pawpaw) is also good eaten whole with a little lemon juice.

Taste test: ✺ ✺ ✺ ✺ ✺
Mellow with a pleasant spiciness; thick and creamy.

Ingredients
✺ 1 papaya (pawpaw), deseeded
✺ 2 green (tart) apples
✺ 4 cm/1½ in root ginger
✺ 1 tbsp ground flaxseeds
  or organic dehulled hemp seeds
✺ 1 tsp cinnamon
✺ ½ cup unsweetened Greek yoghurt
✺ Squeeze of lemon juice
✺ An ice cube

Core and slice the apples and
peel and slice the root ginger,
then blend with the rest of
the ingredients.

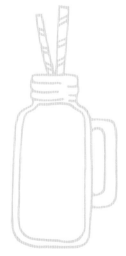

My verdict: ☐☐☐☐☐

DR MAX GERSON

The German raw food pioneer Dr Max Gerson cured cancer patients using chiefly the freshly made raw juices of fruits and vegetables high in potassium and other minerals. He also treated the great philosopher Albert Schweitzer, a severe diabetic taking huge doses of insulin, with a strict protein-free diet and a regime of raw and juiced fruit and vegetables. Despite their high sugar content, apples were also included in this treatment. After only one month on this specialised diet, Schweitzer needed no insulin at all and remained active and healthy until his death in 1956 at the age of 92.

Caribbean Calypso F

Health benefits: Cinnamon is an excellent spice to use to balance blood sugar, and just a small amount can go a long way. Adding coconut milk as the liquid base for the smoothie will help to control blood sugar levels by providing a healthy fat source and balancing out the sugars from the fruit. Bring on the steel band!

Taste test: ✳ ✳ ✳ ✳ ✳
Creamy and tangy with exotic flavours.

SERVES **1–2**

Ingredients
✳ ¼ pineapple, peeled
✳ 1 mango, stoned (pitted) and peeled
✳ ½ tsp ground cinnamon
✳ Coconut milk to the water (max) line
✳ 200 g ice

Combine all the ingredients in the above order in the blender and blend until smooth.

My verdict: ☐ ☐ ☐ ☐ ☐

OCCASIONAL TREATS

Crème de Menthe Indulgence F

Health benefits: The cream in this dessert smoothie makes it a bit of an indulgence but when you're entertaining friends, or want something a bit special, this recipe is quick, easy and delicious. The same recipe can be adapted using strawberries and Crème de Fraise, raspberries and Crème de Framboise, blackcurrant and Cassis, or cherries with Cherry Brandy or Cointreau. Crème de Menthe is good for the digestion and whichever fruit you choose will provide you with a good amount of vitamin C.

Taste test: ✹ ✹ ✹ ✹ ✹
Delectable!

SERVES **4**

Ingredients
- ✹ 250 g green seedless grapes
- ✹ 3 tbsp/¼ cup Crème de Menthe
- ✹ 3 meringues nests, about 65 g/2½ oz
- ✹ 125 ml/½ cup single/light cream
- ✹ 250 ml/1 cup unsweetened almond milk
- ✹ 4 mint leaves
- ✹ 2 ice cubes
- ✹ A mint leaf and a sliced green grape, to garnish
- ✹ (NB Instead of the single cream and almond milk, you can substitute this with 4 scoops of vanilla ice)

Blend all the ingredients together, and serve in coupe glasses or large wine glasses, with an After Eight chocolate wafer!

My verdict: ☐ ☐ ☐ ☐ ☐

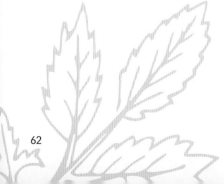

Chocolate Strawberry Dream **F**

Health benefits: Raw, unprocessed cacao is loaded with magnesium, antioxidants and brain-stimulating chemicals that help the body absorb calcium, fight disease and stabilise moods. Strawberries are good for stress, anxiety and irritability and will also help with your memory.

Taste test: ✱ ✱ ✱ ✱ ✱
Strawberry milkshake at its best!

SERVES **2**

Ingredients
- ✱ 2 tbsp of dark chocolate chips or cacao nibs
- ✱ 250 g/8 oz strawberries
- ✱ 125 ml/4½ fl oz whole milk
- ✱ 150 ml/ 5 fl oz fat-free yoghurt
- ✱ 125 ml/4½ fl oz mineral water
- ✱ 8 ice cubes

Place all the ingredients in the blender and blend until smooth. Makes two glasses.

My verdict: ☐ ☐ ☐ ☐ ☐

IMPROVING HEALTH

3. Smoothies for weight loss

'My vegetable love should grow vaster than empires and more slow.'

Andrew Marvell (1622–1678)

The problem with being overweight

According to data from the 2014 Health Survey for England, 62 per cent of the adult population of the UK is overweight or obese. Ordinary slimming diets are notoriously poor nutritionally, and diets of cooked foods, vitamin pills and food supplements will never be as beneficial to your system as raw juice dieting.

According to Cancer Research UK, one in 20 UK cancers are linked to being overweight or obese. Carrying extra fat in the body, especially around the waist, can have harmful effects like producing hormones and growth factors that affect the way our cells work. This can raise the risk of several diseases including cancer. Research has shown that many types of cancer are more common in people who are overweight or obese, including: breast, bowel, oesophageal, stomach, pancreatic, kidney and liver cancer. Being overweight may also contribute to gall bladder, aggressive prostate and ovarian cancer.

The World Cancer Research Fund encourages eating low-calorie, nutrient-rich foods such as fruits, vegetables, grain cereals and pulses as alternatives to calorie-laden, high-fat foods. The juices of fruits and vegetables can be a very important part of such a programme.

Successful dieting

A planned smoothie diet to achieve a desirable body weight can be organised alongside a balanced calorie intake and physical activity. Successful slimming is not achieved overnight but is a long-term process. To be effective, weight loss should be slow and gradual. Dieters who stop and start diets all the time often end up with their bodies containing a higher proportion of body fat than when they first started dieting. This has been called the 'yo-yo' effect', and may be more harmful to health than being slightly overweight. Weight loss should mean losing fat and not other body stores, such as protein from the muscles, but as fat is the body's long-term storage it is the hardest energy store to reduce.

How many calories should we consume?

The Department of Health recommends that an average woman requires approximately 1,940 calories a day, and a man requires approximately 2,550 calories a day to maintain weight. However some recent research suggests that these levels may be too high and some normal-weight women require only 1,850 calories, with the same decreased proportion for men. Studies of overweight people show that the majority of women lose weight on a 1,000–1,200 calorie diet and most men lose weight on 1,200–1,500 calories a day. An excellent target is a loss of 0.45–0.9 kg/1–2 lb per week. This is the equivalent of 500–1,000 calories less than would normally be eaten a day.

Taking regular exercise

It is now recognised that exercise is almost as important as the diet itself. Exercise certainly speeds the process and tones up the muscles, which ultimately improves body shape and increases the suppleness, stamina and strength of the body. People forget that the heart is a muscle and like most muscles needs exercise.

Exercise need not be over-strenuous initially. Regular aerobic classes, swimming, walking, running, jogging, dancing, cycling and digging the garden are all good forms of exercise.

The Department of Health recommendations are that adults (aged 19–24) should aim to be active daily. Over a week, activity should add up to at least 150 minutes (2½ hours) of moderate intensity activity in bouts of 10 minutes or more – one way to approach this is to do 30 minutes on at least five days a week. Alternatively, comparable benefits can be achieved through 75 minutes of vigorous intensity activity spread across the week or combinations of moderate and vigorous intensity activity. Adults should also undertake physical activity to improve muscle strength on at least two days a week and should minimise the amount of time spent being sedentary (sitting) for extended periods.

Fad diets

Remember that the slimming business is a very profitable one. Unfortunately, only a minority of diets are sensible and even these often do not succeed; some fad diets are nutritionally inadequate as they do not provide enough vitamins and minerals; and some even constitute a health risk. Fasting and very severe dieting can cause nausea, vomiting, fatigue, dizziness and low blood pressure and even lead to severe depression and irritability. Unbalanced diets have been criticised by orthodox doctors and dieticians: for example, a highly dangerous liquid protein diet combined with fasting in the 1970s in the USA was believed to have caused at least 60 deaths.

Sticking to your diet

Dieting can be easy to start but sometimes difficult to keep up, and success is possible only if your new way of eating becomes part of a permanent change in lifestyle. Set yourself realistic goals: if you need to shed two stones, concentrate on the first stone before tackling the next. Learn to say a polite no to food outside your diet plan that is offered to you. Try to be hungry at mealtimes, and if you aren't hungry at mealtimes eat a bit less, or perhaps have a little extra at the next meal. There will be times when you want to cheat, but try to keep occupied: some slimmers brush their teeth every time they want to eat, chat to a friend, or find other ways to entertain or distract themselves. You need to discover what triggers your desire to cheat and then develop strategies to deal with those triggers so you don't end up cheating.

Only weigh yourself once or twice a week because your weight fluctuates through the day due to changes in water retention, and disappointing readings can be discouraging. After you have been dieting for a while your weight may seem to remain stationary; this happens as your body gets used to receiving less food and adjusts by slowing your metabolism.

Why not wean your partner from some of those calorie-packed business lunches and offer instead a flask of a freshly made fruit or vegetable smoothie, with perhaps a wholemeal sandwich. The evening meal will be appreciated far more and he or she will be happier and healthier for having shed a few pounds. Simply place an ice cube in the thermos, freshly blend a smoothie and fill the flask to the very top, ready for a snack or picnic!

What is the smoothie diet?

As with any weight reduction diet, it is advisable to check with your doctor before beginning a regime that includes a lot of juices.

Consuming raw fruit and vegetable smoothies in order to slim does not mean starvation but is a great way to lose weight naturally without feeling deprived of food. It means super nutrition and, with regular exercise, it is a safe, slow, steady way to achieve permanent weight loss. It has been said that the same raw food diet prescribed in the health clinics of Europe to treat cancer, diabetes and arthritis can work wonders for the overweight. Health farms continue to heal and rejuvenate their clients with fresh smoothies, but at a price: a blender in your kitchen can provide the same benefits and at far less expense.

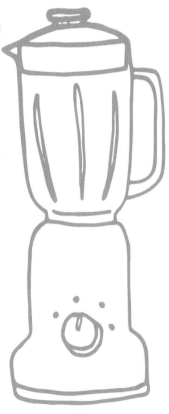

'Living' foods vibrate – giving you a sense of well-being – and fresh smoothies provide you with instant raw energy, a tonic 'pick me up'. The late Dr Norman Walker also said that dieting on smoothies gives you the highest density of nutrients for calorie intake and the lowest fat intake of any diet, and it is the easiest, most comfortable way to lose a few pounds. When overtaxed by stress and obesity, smoothies restore normal responsiveness to the adrenal glands, improve your muscle tone and, most importantly, process the entire body through a spring cleaning, giving your digestive machine a chance to rest.

Simply substitute a smoothie for one of your daily meals, say lunch, and eat your regular breakfast and dinner menu. This way you should lose 2–4 kg/4–8 lb a month. Weight gain can happen over several years and it is, therefore, very wise to slim slowly with a sensible diet. Consuming fruit and vegetable smoothies softens the pangs of hunger and once embarked on this programme for slimming your desire for fattening and sweet foods will disappear. You can always dilute pure fruit juice with a little water to reduce its acidity.

Smoothies that contain carrot, spinach, beetroot (red beet) and cucumber juices are especially recommended for a slimming programme.

The following pages offer 14 delicious and appetising smoothies so you can incorporate two different recipes per day for each day of the week as part of any slimming plan. It is advisable when weight watching not to exceed more than six glasses (500 ml) a day, because large quantities of unsweetened fruit juice shouldn't be drunk on a diet. If you have diabetes, remember to not drink more than 300 ml/day. A 250 ml/8 fl oz fruit smoothie contains about 100 calories and a vegetable smoothie about half that amount.

The calorie content of a fruit smoothie in a small glass (100 ml/3 ½ fl oz) is approximately 50 kilocalories, therefore 1 litre/1 ¾ pt of a blended fruit smoothie would contain approximately 500 kilocalories – which is half a day's calorie allowance for slimmers.

LOSING WEIGHT

Recipes for weight loss

All the smoothies in this section are low in calories and are therefore of great benefit to those trying to lose weight. But don't feel you have to miss out if counting the calories is not your main goal. Just like in the previous chapter, you will find recipes excellent for cleansing the liver and kidneys, aiding digestion, lowering cholesterol, improving your sex life and protecting the body against heart disease and cancer.

Aloha Delight F

Health benefits: This drink is very high in vitamin C, excellent for cleansing the liver and kidneys.

Taste test: ✹ ✹ ✹ ✹ ✹
This pinky-red beauty is a perfect combination of sweet and sour that is mouth-wateringly good.

SERVES **1**

Ingredients
✹ 1 pineapple round, 2.5 cm/1 in thick
✹ ½ sweet eating (dessert) apple
✹ 8 strawberries

Remove and discard the skin of the pineapple and cut the flesh into strips. Cut the apple into wedges. Hull the strawberries and process all the fruits in the blender.

My verdict: ☐ ☐ ☐ ☐ ☐

Weight Watcher's Wonder V/F

Health benefits: As all weight watchers know, celery is a reducing aid. But it is also said to be good for nervous disorders, insomnia and muscle cramping so this is a great drink for athletes and sportsmen.

Taste test: ✹ ✹ ✹

A little watery for my liking but with an astringent taste.

SERVES **1**

Ingredients
- ✳ 2 celery stalks
- ✳ 1 sweet eating (dessert) apple
- ✳ 4 sprigs of parsley (optional)
- ✳ ½ cup/75 ml mineral water
- ✳ ½ tsp fine sea salt or ground Himalayan salt

Cut the celery into 5–7.5cm/2–3 in pieces. Core the apple and cut into narrow wedges. Process all through the blender.

My verdict: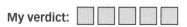

Melon Medley F

Health benefits: Melons are full of vitamins and nutrients. Cantaloupe melons are especially good for you, with beta-carotene levels reported as high as 1765 ug per l00 g/4 oz. They are good for the skin and the nerves and have a tonic effect on digestion.

Taste test: ✳ ✳ ✳ ✳ ✳
Sweet, delicate flavours with added kick; cool and refreshing.

SERVES **1**

Ingredients
- ✳ ¼ cantaloupe melon
- ✳ ¼ watermelon
- ✳ ¼ honeydew melon
- ✳ 1.5 cm/½ in piece of ginger root (optional)
- ✳ 1 ice cube

Cut up and dice all the melons removing their seeds and skins. Add the sliced ginger root, and blend all together with the ice cube in the blender.

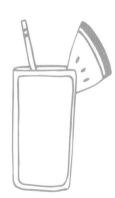

My verdict:

Top 'n' Tail Tonic **V/F**

Health benefits: Carrot juice has a very high content of beta-carotene, vitamin C and B-complex vitamins and many valuable minerals. The carbohydrates in carrots give you energy and they are good for the lymphatic system, the blood, the skin, vision and digestion, so juicing carrots should be very much part of your everyday diet right from the start. The celery in this recipe is a rich source of organic sodium and therefore relieves muscle cramping. Parsley is a great blood purifier.

Taste test: ✳ ✳ ✳
Pleasant, nutty and spicy, a bit like celery soup.

SERVES **1**

Ingredients
- ✳ 2 carrots
- ✳ 1 celery stick
- ✳ ½ sweet apple
- ✳ 4 sprigs of parsley
- ✳ 1 ice cube

Trim the carrots and cut into 5–7.5 cm/2–3 in pieces. Cut the celery into pieces. Core and cut the apple into narrow wedges. Process all the vegetables and apple through the blender with the ice cube.

My verdict: ☐ ☐ ☐ ☐ ☐

LOSING WEIGHT

Pineapple Paradise **F**

Health benefits: Grapefruit contains bioflavonoids, especially naringin which thins the blood and lowers cholesterol. Pink grapefruit has as much vitamin C as oranges and is high in beta-carotene, which protects against heart disease and cancer and boosts the immune system.

Taste test: ✳ ✳ ✳ ✳ ✳
A tongue-tingling, exotic blend of sweet and sour.

SERVES **1**

Ingredients

* 1 pineapple round, 2.5 cm/1 in thick
* ½ pink grapefruit
* ½ sweet eating (dessert) apple
* 1 ice cube

Remove and discard the skin of the pineapple and cut the flesh into strips. Peel the grapefruit, leaving on as much white pith as possible. Cut the apple into narrow wedges. Process the fruits and ice cube in the blender.

My verdict: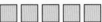

Body Builder **V/F**

Health benefits: By now you will know all about the many health properties in carrots and apples, but cauliflowers are also high in vitamin C and many useful minerals. The apple sweetens this drink, but you could use another carrot instead of the apple.

Taste test:
Pleasantly sweet but earthy.

SERVES **1**

Ingredients

* 2 carrots
* 2 cauliflower florets with stems
* 1 sweet eating (dessert) apple
* 4 sprigs of parsley
* A pinch of fine sea salt
* 1 ice cube

Trim the carrots and cut into 5–7.5 cm/2–3 in pieces. Slice the cauliflower florets and stems into strips. Cut the apple into narrow wedges. Process all through the blender with the ice cube.

My verdict: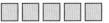

Simply Apple and Pear **F**

Health benefits: Pears contain a lot of pectin, a digestive aid that helps regulate the body. Pears strengthen the kidneys and they are said to be good for sleeplessness.

Taste test: ✳ ✳ ✳ ✳
Pears are beautifully sweet so it's best to choose a tarter variety of apple for this one.

SERVES **1**

Ingredients
✳ 2 tart eating (dessert) apples
✳ 1 pear
✳ 1 ice cube

Core the apples and pear and slice into wedges. Process all through the blender with the ice cube.

My verdict: ☐ ☐ ☐ ☐ ☐

Green Lite **V/F**

Health benefits: Courgettes (zucchinis) are low in calories – only 18 per 100g so ideal for weight reduction. They are a good source of potassium which helps reduce blood pressure. Spinach has many health benefits; it is good for the eyes, builds the bones, aids digestion, eases constipation and flushes toxins from the body,

Taste test: ✳ ✳ ✳
Rehydrating, mellow and light.

SERVES **2**

Ingredients
✳ 115 g/4 oz sliced courgette (zucchini)
✳ 50 g/1¾ oz baby spinach leaves

* 2 apples, peeled, cored and quartered
* Fill to the water line with mineral water
* Sweeten with a little honey if necessary

Place all the ingredients in the blender and blend until smooth.

My verdict: ☐☐☐☐☐

Peach Perfection F

Health benefits: Peaches contain about 35–50 calories and no fat so are excellent for those wanting to lose weight. They are also high in potassium and low in sodium which is good for controlling blood pressure. They are easy on the digestive system, cleanse the kidneys and bladder and help maintain radiant skin. Grapes are also good for the kidneys, colon and heart, and can help with anaemia and soothe the nervous system. If the grapes are sweet enough, the quantity of apple juice can be increased.

Taste test: ✹ ✹ ✹ ✹ ✹
A delectable honey-coloured delight.

SERVES **1**

Ingredients
* 4 oz/115 g red or green
  seedless grapes
* 1 peach, stoned (pitted)
* 1 sweet eating (dessert) apple
* 1 ice cube

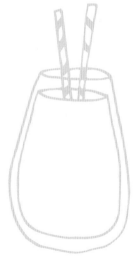

Cut the apple into wedges and place all the fruit and the ice cube through the blender and serve.

My verdict: ☐☐☐☐☐

Tropical Teaser　**F**

Health benefits: Foods with antioxidant properties are those rich in beta-carotene and vitamins C and E and are known to significantly improve our mood. Spinach, pineapple and kale are some of the best antioxidant foods.

Taste test: 🌟 🌟 🌟 🌟 🌟
Wonderfully refreshing with a tasty kick.

SERVES **1**

Ingredients
* 🌟 40 g/1½ oz wheatgrass juice, or handful of spinach or kale
* 🌟 ¼ pineapple, peeled
* 🌟 1.5 cm/½ in piece of root ginger
* 🌟 1 ice cube

Juice the wheatgrass separately if you have a juicer, then blend the pineapple and ginger together with the wheatgrass. Otherwise blend the pineapple and ginger along with the spinach or kale.

My verdict: ☐ ☐ ☐ ☐ ☐

Fennel Fusion　**V**

Health benefits: This is a colourful drink and very good for the bloodstream. Beetroot (red beet) contains many minerals, and it is a tremendous aid to the liver and gall bladder. It's potent, so you must only juice a little and dilute it with apple juice or sparkling mineral water. The fennel aids digestion.

Taste test: 🌟 🌟 🌟 🌟 🌟
The strong liquorice flavour of the fennel hides the rather earthy taste of the beetroot (red beet), resulting in a truly delicious and nutritious combo.

SERVES **1**

Ingredients

* 1 small fennel bulb (approx. 100 g/4 oz)
* ¼ beetroot (red beet)
* 3 apples

Cut the fennel and beetroot (red beet) into narrow wedges. Core the apples and cut into narrow wedges and process them through the blender. If the mixture is too thick for your liking, thin it down with some mineral water.

My verdict: ☐☐☐☐☐

Aphrodite's Love Potion F

Health benefits: Certain foods have been recommended for provoking erotic desire for centuries, particularly by the Ancient Greek and Roman civilisations. Some fruits play their part in provoking desire: those that are rich in vitamins A and E and zinc are said to improve your sex life.

Taste test: ✸ ✸ ✸ ✸ ✸
A coral-coloured elixir; creamy, sweet and very delicious.

SERVES **1**

Ingredients

* 1 mango
* 1 pineapple round, 2.5 cm/1 in thick
* 6 strawberries
* 1 ice cube

Halve the mango and remove the stone (pit). Cut the flesh away from the skin. Cut the flesh into strips. Remove and discard the skin of the pineapple and cut the flesh into strips. Hull the strawberries. Blend all the fruits together.

My verdict: ☐☐☐☐☐

Garlic Guardian V

Health benefits: Garlic, a good source of potassium, has for many years had a reputation as a miracle cure for all kinds of ills. It has now been medically proven as an antiseptic and antifungal agent, and it helps to prevent blood clots and lowers blood cholesterol levels. It also destroys free radicals, so it is a cancer fighter. Experts believe that one or two cloves a day are enough for protection.

Taste test: ✴ ✴ ✴ ✴
If you like garlic bread, you'll love this!

SERVES **1**

Ingredients
✴ 2 carrots
✴ A handful of parsley
✴ 1 garlic clove
✴ 2 celery sticks or a slice of fennel
✴ 1 cup/250 ml mineral water or coconut water

Trim the carrots and cut them into 5–7.5 cm/2–3 in pieces. Place all the vegetables through the blender.

My verdict: ☐ ☐ ☐ ☐ ☐

LOSING WEIGHT

Italian Serenade V

Health benefits: It is said that there is more than 50 per cent of the RDA of vitamin C in one tomato. Half a cucumber juiced instead of the apple juice also makes a good combination.

Taste test: ✴ ✴ ✴ ✴
Sweet and aromatic with flavours of the Mediterranean.

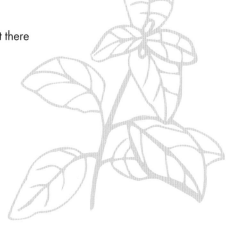

Ingredients

- ✳ 2 large vine-ripened tomatoes
- ✳ 1 Golden Delicious apple
- ✳ 3 basil leaves (more, if wished), chopped
- ✳ A small slice of lime
- ✳ A pinch of fine sea salt or ground Himalayan salt (optional)
- ✳ Crushed ice
- ✳ Basil leaves, to garnish

Cut the tomatoes and apple into small wedges. Process in the blender with the basil leaves and lime. Pour over crushed ice, garnish with bruised basil leaves and serve.

My verdict: ☐ ☐ ☐ ☐ ☐

4. Smoothies for specific conditions

'No illness that can be treated by diet should be treated by any other means.'

Maimonedes, twelfth-century Jewish physician

Now you have made a start at including smoothies as part of your diet, you can create your own recipes and add other ingredients, particularly if you have specific conditions you want to target.

The following tables have been compiled after careful research and interviews with health professionals. The responsive conditions mentioned are merely a guide to remedies and their therapeutic benefits to general health and, are NOT intended to replace medical advice: only a trained physician can diagnose and treat serious illness.

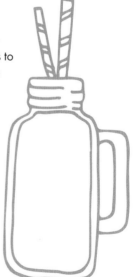

All the ingredients listed, however, can provide you with healthy and enjoyable nourishment as part of any diet plan that incorporates smoothies.

A–Z of juicing ingredients with their benefits

Fruit	Vitamins	Minerals	Juicy extras	Good for…	Extra benefits	Preparation
apple	C	potassium	malic acid, nectin, ellagic acid, high in soluble fibre	acne, anaemia, arthritis, asthma, circulatory weakness, constipation, convalescence, cystitis, diabetes, diarrhoea, eczema, fever, gout, haemorrhoids, headache and migraine, indigestion, kidney and liver disorders, menopause, menstrual problems, nausea, prostate, respiratory problems, rheumatism, sciatica, weight loss	good for blood sugar and lowering cholestrol levels	slice in half, remove core, seeds and stem
apricot	beta-carotene, C	copper, sodium, potassium	rich in antioxidant; good source of fibre; anti-imflammatory	anaemia, blood pressure control, cancer (prostate), constipation, fever, sciatica, skin disorders	helps protect your eyes from age-related damage; promotes healthy hair and skin	cut in half, remove stone (pit)
bananas	B6, beta-carotene, biotin, C, folic acid	copper, magnesium, manganese, potassium, sodium		anaemia, asthma, blood pressure, constipation, depression, diabetes, diarrhoea, digestion, eye disorders, menstrual problems, muscle cramps, nausea, pregnancy and childbirth, stress, ulcers	promotes a healthy heart	remove skin and break into two or three sections

continued ▶

blackberry	A, C, E, folate, K	potassium	high in fibre; high in antioxidants especially anthocyanin and ellagic acid	blood pressure, circulatory weakness, diarrhoea, menopause, pregnancy and childbirth, skin disorders	helps memory loss; maintains eye, heart and digestive health; prevents blood vessel damage	wash and use as is
blackcurrant	beta-carotene, C, E	calcium, magnesium	high in antioxidants especially anthocyanin	bladder disorders, cancer, circulatory weakness, convalescence, cystitis, eczema, heart disease, menopause, respiratory problems, sore throat, urinary tract disorder	the rich level of vitamin C is a protection against cancer and heart disease	wash and use as is
blueberry	beta-carotene, C, folic acid, K	copper, calcium, iron, magnesium, manganese, phosphorus, potassium, sodium, zinc	high in fibre; high in flavonoids; antioxidant and anti-inflammatory	acne, bladder disorders, blood pressure, cancer (colon), diarrhoea, insomnia, impotence, joint pain, kidney and liver disorders, sciatica, thyroid disorders, varicose veins, urinary tract infection	improves memory; helps lower LDL levels; helps with muscle recovery after strenuous exercise	wash and use as is
cherry	A	magnesium, phosphorous, potassium		anaemia, arthritis, catarrh, constipation, cramps, gallstones, gout, indigestion, impotence, menstrual problems, prostate disorders, rheumatism, sciatica, urinary tract disorder, weight loss		remove stalk and discard the stones (pit) using a cherry stoner

	Vitamins	Minerals	Properties	Conditions	Benefits	Preparation
cranberry	A, B6, C, E, K, pantothnic acid	copper, manganese, phosphorus	high in fibre; high in the phytonutrient quercetin which is a potent antioxidant and anti-inflammatory	asthma, bladder disorders, cystitis, cancer (breast, colon, lung and prostate), colds and flu, diarrhoea, fever, fluid retention, kidney disorders, lung disorders, prostate disorders, skin disorders, stomach ulcers, urinary tract infection, weight loss		wash and use as is
dates	A, B6, K	potassium, iron, copper, magnesium, niacin	high in dietary fibre	anaemia, arthritis, blood pressure, cancer (breast, colon, lung, prostate), colitis, constipation, diarrhoea, eye disorders, impotence, lung disorders, menopause, pregnancy, respiratory problems, weight loss	helps maintain healthy heart	remove stone (pit)
goji berries	C, E	calcium, potassium and up to 21 trace minerals	contain 500 times the vitamin C content per weight of oranges; high in fibre	arthritis, blood pressure, colds and flu, eye problems, heart health, kidney and liver disorders, skin disorders, weight loss		wash and use as is
grape	A, B2, C, K, niacin	copper, potassium	tartaric acid	anaemia, anxiety, blood disorders, blood pressure, cancer (breast, colon, prostate), catarrh, constipation, fever, gout, haemorrhoids, heart health, indigestion, kidney disorders, liver disorders, menstrual problems, rheumatism, skin disorders, stress, weight loss	grapes stimulate kidney function and help regulate the heartbeat; they cleanse the liver and eliminate uric acid from the body; they soothe the nervous system	remove from stem

grapefruit	A, B, biotin, B1, C, pantothenic acid	potassium	high in fibre; lycopenes and liminoids act as antioxidants; salicylic acid, pectin	cancer (prostate), catarrh, colds, coughs, ear disorders, fatigue, fever, gout, halitosis, hangover, hay fever, indigestion, insomnia, liver disorders, menopause, pregnancy, pyorrhoea, skin disorders, sore throat, varicose veins, weight loss	pink and red grapefruit are high in lycopenes which help fight prostate cancer Be aware of grapefruit and certain drug interactions: speak with your doctor	peel but leave as much pith on as you can
kiwi fruit	A, B6, C, E, K	magnesium, manganese, phosphorus, potassium	high in fibre; phytochemical: lutein	catarrh, circulatory weakness, colds and flu, coughs, digestive weakness, fatigue, high blood pressure, skin disorders, sore throat, stress, weight loss	promotes healthy eyes and heart	peel off skin
lemon/lime	B6, C, folate	potassium	bioflavonoids, citric acid	anaemia, arthritis, asthma, cancer, catarrh, colds, constipation, coughs, cystitis, digestive disorders, ear disorders, fever, fluid retention, gout, hair loss, halitosis, hangover, indigestion, infection, insomnia, kidney stones, liver disorders, nausea, nervous disorders, pneumonia, pyorrhoea, rheumatism, skin disorders, sore throat, varicose veins, weight loss	lemon juice protects the mucous membranes lining the digestive tract; helps immune function	remove the skin

mango	A, beta-carotene, B1, B6, C, E,	copper, potassium	high in fibre	acne, blood pressure, cancer (breast, colon, leukemia, prostate), constipation, eye health, hangover, indigestion, kidney disorders, liver disorders, sciatica, sinusitis, ulcers, weight loss	NB people who take warfarin need to be aware of the effects of consuming mango – consult your doctor	halve the fruit horizontally, remove the large stone (pit), then strip off the tough outer skin
melon (all varieties)	A, B6, C, folic acid	copper, magnesium, phosphorus, potassium		anxiety, arthritis, bladder disorders, constipation, cramps, cystitis, fluid retention, headache and migraine, kidney disorders, mouth ulcers, prostate disorders, skin disorders, stress, varicose veins, weight loss	they are cooling and have a tonic effect on digestion	discard the seeds and peel
nectarine	A, B1, B2, B6, C, niacin	magnesium, phosphorus, potassium		blood pressure, heart problems, weight loss	maintains healthy skin and eyes	remove the stone (pit) and juice the whole fruit
orange	A, biotin, C, folic acid, niacin; small amounts of B1, B2, B6, E and K	calcium, iron, potassium, phosphorus, zinc	inositol, bioflavonoids and 11 amino acids	anaemia, asthma, blood disorders, cancer, catarrh, colds, coughs, diabetes, fatigue, fever, gout, halitosis, hangover, hay fever, heart disease, high blood pressure, indigestion, liver disorders, lung disorders, menopause, pneumonia, pyorrhoea, rheumatism, skin disorders, sore throat, weight loss	cleanses and tones the gastrointestinal tract. The heart and lungs also benefit, and overly acidic blood is alkalised by drinking orange juice on a regular basis	peel off the skin but leave as much pith as you can

continued ▶

SPECIFIC
CONDITIONS

papaya (pawpaw)	A, beta-carotene, C	copper, magnesium, potassium	laevulose; high in fibre	acne, arthritis, blood disorders, cancer (colon), colds and flu, constipation, coughs, diabetes, eczema, eye health, gout, heart health, immune function, indigestion, kidney disorders, liver disorders, sciatica, sore throat, tumours, ulcers, weight loss	contains laevulose, especially suitable for diabetics; contains an active principle called papain, which is of considerable value in dyspepsia and helps to digest protein	discard the seeds and peel
peach	A (beta-carotene), B3, C, E, niacin	iron, potassium		blood disorders, constipation, diabetes, indigestion, morning sickness, pregnancy and childbirth	the juice cleanses the intestines and stimulates activity in the lower bowel	remove the stone (pit) and juice the whole fruit
pear	C, K	copper, phosphorus, potassium	pectin, fibre	bladder disorders, constipation, insomnia, liver disorders, prostate disorders	the pectin in pears is a valued aid to digestion; pears cleanse the body of toxins and other waste by stimulating bowel activity	buy firm but ripe pears for juicing

pineapple	A, B1, B6, B-complex, C, E, folate, pantothetic acid	calcium, copper, iron, manganese, sodium, phosphorus, potassium	bromeline, fibre	anxiety, blood disorders, colds, depression, digestive problems, gout, hangover, indigestion, kidney disorders, menopause, menstrual problems, muscular problems, pneumonia, pyorrhoea, sciatica, sore throat, stress, weight loss	bromeline in pineapples helps to balance and neutralise fluids that are either too alkaline or too acidic, and also stimulates hormonal secretion in the pancreas	choose pineapples with a yellow skin, that smell strong and sweet, and give a little when pressed; remove the skin
plum	C, E, K	calcium, iron, magnesium, potassium	malic acid	bladder disorders, circulatory weakness, constipation, fatigue		remove stones (pits) and dilute the thick juice with water or apple or grape juice
pomegranate	B5, B6, C, folate, K	manganese phosphorus, potassium, sodium	fibre, phytochemicals	cancer (prostate), constipation, cystitis, high blood pressure, menopause	Helps lower cholesterol; promotes dental, digestive and heart health; aids recovery after exercise	cut fruit in half, bang the outer skin with a spoon to loosen the seeds; remove skin

continued ▶

	Vitamins	Minerals	Other	Conditions	Benefits	Preparation
prunes and dried fruit	A, B6, K	copper, iron, magnesium, potassium	benzoic and quinic acid, soluble fibre, sorbitol	anaemia, arthritis, constipation, haemorrhoids, heart health, weight loss	promotes healthy bones; controls blood sugar	soak 15 stoned (pitted) prunes overnight in 1.2 litres/2 pt/5 cups of hot water, then blend in a blender with the soaking water; strain the juice and discard the pulp
raspberry	B5, C, E, folate, K	calcium, iron, magnesium, manganese, potassium	ellagic acid, fibre	circulatory weakness, convalescence, digestive disorders, fatigue, fever, nervous tension, thyroid disorders		wash and use as is
strawberry	beta-carotene, C, folate	manganese	antioxidant, anti-inflammatory, ellagic acid	acne, anxiety, blood pressure, constipation, fever, fluid retention, gout, hay fever, indigestion, kidney disorders, menopause, motion sickness, nausea, pneumonia, prostate disorders, pyorrhoea, rheumatism, stress, thyroid disease, weight loss	highly cleansing to the blood, tissues and muscles; promotes heart health and nerve function	wash strawberries thoroughly, and remove the green stalks

Vegetables and herbs	Vitamins	Minerals	Juicy extras	Good for...	Extra benefits	Use and preparation
avocado	beta-carotene, B6, C, E, folate, K, pantothenic acid (B5)	calcium, copper, iron, magnesium, manganese, phosphorus, potassium	essential natural good fats – monounsaturated fat; high in fibre; high antioxidant and anti-inflammatory phytonutrients	arthritis, blood pressure, bone problems, constipation, cramps, depression, diabetes, digestion, eye disorders, hangover, headache and migraine, heart health, kidney problems, liver disorders, thrush, weight loss	helps control blood sugar; good for the heart	cut in half, twist, remove stone (pit), scrape out flesh from skin
basil	A, C, folate, K	calcium, copper, magnesium, manganese		arthritis, asthma, heart health, IBS, Inflammatory bowel disease, joint problems, osteoarthritis	anti-bacterial properties	wash and use as is

continued ▶

	Vitamins	Minerals	Other	Conditions	Benefits	Use
beetroot (red beet)	A, B6, C, folic acid	calcium, chlorine, chromium, copper, iron, magnesium, manganese, phosphorus, potassium, sodium	phytonutrients betanin and vulgaxanthins provide antioxidant and anti-inflammatory support; fibre	acne, anaemia, arthritis, bladder, disorders, cancer (colon), circulatory weakness, colitis, cystitis, depression, diarrhoea, eczema, fatigue, fever, hangover, high blood pressure, impotence, kidney disorders, liver disorders, laryngitis, menopause, menstrual problems, muscular problems, nervous disorders, prostate disorders, rheumatism, skin disorders, thrush, urinary tract disorder; weight loss	very powerful detox cleanser and builder of the blood; promotes eye and heart health	use moderately – 50 g/2 oz of beetroot (red beet) juice mixed with 175 g/6 oz of apple, carrot or cucumber juice is ample
broccoli	A, beta-carotene, B2, B6, C, E, folic acid, K, pantothenic acid	calcium, chromium, copper, iron, manganese, phosphorus, potassium, sulphur	fibre	anxiety, cancer, circulatory weakness, cystitis, depression, fatigue, hangover, indigestion, insomnia, joint problems, motion sickness, nausea, sciatica, stress, thrush, varicose veins	contains sulforaphane, which has anti-cancer properties	mix with other vegetables to improve flavour
cabbage	A (as beta-carotene), B6, C, folate, K, niacin	manganese, potassium	antioxidants, anti-inflamatory, fibre	asthma, bladder disorders, blood pressure disorders, bronchitis, circulatory weakness, colitis, constipation, digestive problems, fatigue, fever, hair loss, halitosis, hangover, kidney and liver problems, mouth ulcers, pyorrhoea, skin disorders, stress, thrush, ulcers	very good for stomach ulcers	mix with other vegetables especially carrot; cut head into 1 to 2 in wedges

carrot	A, B6, beta-carotene, biotin, C, D, E, K	, calcium, chromium, iron, magnesium, molybdenum, phosphorus, potassium, sodium, sulphur	fibre, carotenoids	acne, anaemia, anxiety, arthritis, asthma, bladder problems, bone problems, cancer, cataracts, circulatory weakness, cystitis, depression, diabetes, diarrhoea, digestive weakness, eczema, eye disorders, gout, haemorrhoids, hair loss, halitosis, hangover, insomnia, kidney disorders, laryngitis, liver disorders, menopause, mouth ulcers, muscular weakness, nervous disorders, prostate disorders, rheumatism, respiratory disorders, sciatica, sinusitis, skin disorders, stress, thrush, ulcers, varicose veins, weight loss	promotes healthy eyes, skin, hair and nails; reduces cholesterol	scrub skin and cut into 1 in chunks
cauliflower	B6, biotin, C, folate, K, pantothenic acid	choline, manganese, phosphorous, potassium	fibre, phytonutrients providing antioxidant and anti-inflammatory support	cancer, fatigue	aids in detoxification	best combined with carrots or apples; outer leaves should be springy

continued ▶

celery	B-complex, beta-carotene, C, E, K	calcium, iron, magnesium, molybdenum, potassium, sodium, sulphur		anxiety, asthma, bronchitis, cancer, circulatory weakness, constipation, cramps, cystitis, diabetes, diarrhoea, eye disorders, fatigue, fluid retention, gout, hangover, headache and migraine, indigestion, insomnia, kidney disorders, liver disorders, menopause, mouth ulcers, muscular problems, nervous disorders, prostate disorders, rheumatism, stress, thrush, weight loss	has a calming effect on nervous conditions and is good for weight-reducing diets; cleanses the body of carbon dioxide	break stalks off from base, cut off bottoms; use leafy tops if fresh
courgette (zucchini)	A, B-complex, C, folates	iron,: manganese, phosphorus, potassium, zinc		arthritis, asthma, bladder disorders, blood pressure problems, constipation, eye disorders, heart problems, muscular problems, pregnancy and childbirth, prostate, weight loss	acts as an internal body brush, cleansing the whole system	cut off ends
cucumber	A, B, beta-carotene, C, K	silica, sodium, magnesium, manganese, phosphorus, potassium	lignans, flavonoids	acne, arthritis, bladder disorders, circulatory weakness, constipation, cystitis, eczema, fatigue, fever, fluid retention, hair loss, halitosis, hangover, high blood pressure, kidney and liver disorders, laryngitis, muscular problems, prostate disorders, rheumatism, scaly skin disorders, thrush, weight loss	good for complexion, may promote hair and fingernail growth; natural diuretic	cut off ends; leave skin on if organic and unwaxed; discard if not

fennel	B3, C, folate, pantothenic acid	calcium, iron, magnesium, manganese, molybdenum, phosphorus, potassium, sodium		arthritis, bone problems, bronchitis, digestive problems, gout, headache and migraine, kidney disorders, liver disorders, menstrual problems, nervous disorders, skin disorders, weight loss	contains an essential oil soothing to an irritated stomach; especially good for the nerves	cut off the base of the bulb; chop the rest into 2 in pieces
garlic	B6, C	copper, iodine, iron, magnesium, manganese, phosphorus, potassium, selenium	allicin	anxiety, asthma, blood pressure disorders, bronchitis, cancer (stomach), circulatory weakness, depression, fatigue, fever, headache and migraine, iron metabolism, joint disorders, liver disorders, respiratory disorders, sinusitis, skin disorders, stress, thrush, urinary tract disorders	lowers the incidence of blood-clotting, boosts the immune system and rids the body of toxins.	skin can be left on
ginger	B2, B3, B6, C,	iron, magnesium, manganese, phosphorus, potassium, zinc		acne, anxiety, arthritis, constipation, eczema, fatigue, fever, halitosis, hangover, headache and migraine, indigestion, lung disorders, nausea, pregnacy and childbirth, prostate disorders, respiratory problems, sinusitis, sore throat, stress, thrush, varicose veins	anti-inflammatory; aids digestion	cut a 1.5–2.5 cm/¼ –½ in piece of root; peel the ginger and grate

continued ▶

Jerusalem artichoke	A, B1, B2, B3, B5, B6, C, folate, K, niacin	iron, magnesium, manganese, phosphorus, potassium, sodium	inutase, inulin, fibre	diabetes, digestion, fatigue, heart disease, hypoglycaemia, IBS, liver disorders, weight loss	good for diabetics as loaded with inulin, an energy source similar to sugar; controls blood sugar	cook lightly
kale	beta-carotene, B1, B2, B3, B6, C, E, folate, K	copper, calcium, iron, magnesium, manganese, phosphorus, potassium	omega-3 fats, fibre, anti-inflammatory, antioxidant, high in nutrients and very low in calories	anaemia, anxiety, arthritis, asthma, cancer, circulatory weakness, cystitis, depression, diabetes, eye disorders, fatigue, hair loss, hangover, hay fever, impotence, liver disorders, motion sickness, muscular problems, nausea, pregnancy and childbirth, skin disorders, stress, thrush, ulcers, weight loss	Can help lower cholesterol	mix with other combinations of vegetables
lettuce	A, B1, B2, B6, C, E, folate, K	chlorophyll, iron, manganese, phosphorus, potassium, silicon		acne, anaemia, constipation, diabetes, hair loss, insomnia, liver disorders, motion sickness, muscular problems, nausea, nervous disorders, prostate disorders, thrush, weight loss	promotes healthy skin and hair; calms the nerves and relaxes the muscles	discard outer limp leaves; use fresh leaves

	vitamins	minerals	active compounds	conditions	properties	notes
mint	A, C	calcium, iron, manganese, potassium, zinc		asthma, cancer, colitis, coughs, halitosis, IBS, indigestion, motion sickness, nausea, stomach ache	anti-bacterial	use leaves and not stems
parsley	A, C, chlorophyll, folate, E, K	calcium, magnesium, manganese, phosphorus, potassium, sodium, sulphur and, especially, iron	luteolin and lycopene provide antioxidant support, apigenin works as an anti-inflammatory	anaemia, anxiety, arthritis, asthma, bladder disorders, bone problems, cancer, circulatory weakness, cystitis, depression, diabetes, diarrhoea, eye disorders, fatigue, gout, headache and migraine, heart disease, insomnia, kidney disorders, liver disorders, lung disorders, menopause, muscular problems, prostate disorders, skin disorders, stress, thrush, urinary tract infection, weight loss	blood and body cleanser, particularly of the kidneys, liver and urinary tract; an aid to good eyesight; avoid excessive consumption if you are pregnant	must be mixed in small amounts with other fruit and vegetables as it is very potent
parsnip	B1, B3, C, folate, K, pantothenic acid, some E	iron, magnesium, manganese, phosphorous, potassium, silicon, sulphur, zinc	insoluble fibre, antioxidants	acne, arthritis, asthma, bladder disorders, bone problems, cancer, cataract, diabetes, digestive weakness, eye disorders, hay fever, liver disorders, muscular weakness, pregnancy and childbirth, sinusitis, skin disorders, ulcers, weight loss	good for the nutrition of the skin, hair and nails	scrub skin and cut into 1 in chunks

continued ▶

	Vitamins	Minerals	Other	Conditions	Action	Notes
peppers (bell peppers)	A (beta-carotene), B1, B6, C (high)	manganese, potassium, silicon	high in lycopenes which act as antioxidants	acne, anxiety, arthritis, circulatory weakness, cystitis, depression, eye disorders, hair loss, heart disease, high blood pressure, kidney disorders, motion sickness, muscular problems, nausea, sciatica, skin disorders, stress, thrush, thyroid disorders, urinary tract disorder	stimulate the circulation and tone and cleanse the arteries and heart muscles	discard stem and seeds
potato	A, B6, C	calcium, copper, iron, magnesium, phosphorus, potassium, manganese, sodium, sulphur	fibre especially if you eat with skin on; antioxidants	arthritis, circulatory weakness, constipation, diarrhoea, digestive disorders, eczema, fatigue, haemorrhoids, muscular problems, peptic ulcers, varicose veins		must be sweetened with honey or diluted with carrot, lemon or apple
seaweed (powder or granules available from most health food shops)		12 key minerals including calcium, iron, magnesium		colds, enlarged adenoids, fatigue, infection, weight loss	stimulates the digestive action of the intestines	sprinkle on to carrot, celery, parsley and spinach smoothies; use no more than 1.5 ml/¼ tsp daily

spinach	A, B1, B2, B3, B6, chlorophyll, E, folate, K, pantothenic acid	calcium, choline, copper, iron, magnesium, manganese, phosphorous, potassium, selenium, sodium, zinc	oxalic acid, fibre	acne, anaemia, anxiety, arthritis, asthma, cancer, circulatory weakness, colitis, constipation, cystitis, depression, diabetes, diarrhoea, digestive weakness, eczema, eye disorders, fatigue, gout, haemorrhoids, hair loss, halitosis, heart problems, high blood pressure, infection, kidney disorders, laryngitis, liver disorders, menopause, motion sickness, mouth ulcers, muscular problems, nausea, nervous disorders, prostate disorders, pyorrhoea, sciatica, skin disorders, stress, thrush, thyroid irregularity, ulcers, varicose veins, weight loss	builds the blood and revitalises constitution	spinach is best used in moderation (i.e. 30 ml/ 2 tbsp) mixed with a combination of other vegetables, preferably carrot, only once or twice a week
tomato	A, biotin, C, E, K	copper, iodine, iron, manganese, molydenum, potassium	lycopenes	anaemia, bladder disorders, depression, diabetes, digestive weakness, gout, hangover, kidney disorders, liver disorders, menopause, prostate, sciatica, sinusitis, skin disorders, stress, thrush, varicose veins, weight loss	highly cleansing to the liver, and good for digestive upsets; good for bone health	remove stalk

continued ▶

	Vitamins	Minerals	Other	Conditions	Properties	Usage
watercress	A, C, K	calcium, iodine, iron		acne, anaemia, asthma, bladder disorders, circulatory weakness, eczema, haemorrhoids, hair loss, intestinal disorders, kidney disorders, liver disorders, lung disorders, menstrual problems, muscular problems, respiratory problems, rheumatism, skin disorders, thyroid irregularity, urinary tract disorders, varicose veins, weight loss	purifier and strengthener of the blood; contains gluconasturtin, which when chewed, chopped or juiced neutralises a carcinogen in tobacco	wash and use as is
wheatgrass	A, beta-carotene, B-complex, C, E, K	calcium, copper, iron, magnesium, manganese, phosphorus, potassium, selenium, zinc	amino acids, chlorophyll, dietary fibre	acne, anaemia, anxiety, arthritis, asthma, bladder disorders, bone disorders, bronchitis, cancer, circulatory weakness, colitis, constipation, cystitis, diabetes, eye disorders, fatigue, hair loss, hay fever, heart disease, high blood pressure, hypoglycaemia, impotence, infection, kidney disorders, liver disorders, low blood pressure, mouth ulcers, nervous disorders, premature ageing, skin disorders, stress, ulcers, weight loss		include in your diet gradually building from 25 g/1 oz to 100 g/4 oz a day.

Nuts, seeds and cereals	Vitamins	Minerals	Extras	Good for…	Extra benefits	Preparation (add to smoothies)
almonds	B2, biotin, E	calcium, copper, iron, magnesium, manganese, phosphorus, potassium	monounsaturated fats, high in fibre	acne, bladder disorders, blood pressure, bone problems, diabetes, fatigue, headache and migraine, heart problems, joint problems, pregnancy and childbirth, rheumatism, sciatica, weight loss	lowers cholesterol and reduces risk of heart disease	if in shell, remove from shell
flaxseeds	B1, B6, folate, K, niacin, thiamin	calcium, copper, iron, magnesium, manganese, phosphorus, potassium, selenium, zinc	rich source of omega-3 fatty acids; high in fibre; antioxidant	acne, bladder disorder, constipation, depression, digestive problems, haemorrhoids, hair loss, joint problems, menopause, sciatica, weight loss		Add 1–3 tbsp of ground flaxseed to your smoothies
oats	B6, E	chromium, copper, magnesium, manganese, phosphorus, selenium, zinc	antioxidant and anti-inflammatory; high in fibre	asthma, bladder disorders, constipation, depression, diabetes fatigue, heart problems, haemorrhoids, infections, menopause	lowers cholesterol; helps control blood sugar; aids digestion	extract as is

continued ▶

SPECIFIC CONDITIONS

peanuts	B3, E, niacin	biotin, copper, manganese, phosphorus	antioxidant; rich in monounsaturated fat	Alzheimer's, anaemia, anxiety, arthritis, bladder disorders, blood pressure problems, bone problems, cancer (colon, stomach), depression, fatigue, gallstones, insomnia, joint problems, menopause, stress, rheumatism, weight loss	helps maintain a healthy heart	extract as is
pumpkin seeds	K	copper, iron, magnesium, manganese, phosphrous, zinc		acne, arthritis, blood pressure, bone problems, constipation, diabetes, headaches and migraines, heart problems, inflammation, insomnia, joint problems, liver problems, menopause, prostate problems, skin problems, stress	promotes healthy eyes	extract as is

sesame seeds	B2, folate, K+, thiamine, tryptophan	calcium, copper, magnesium, manganese, phosphorus, zinc	acne, anaemia, anxiety, arthritis, blood pressure, bone problems, constipation, diabetes, digestive problems, eye disorders, hair loss, heart problems, insomnia, joint problems, liver problems, menopause, respiratory problems, skin problems, stress	lowers cholesterol	extract as is
sunflower seeds	B1, B2, B3, B5, B6, E, folate	calcium, copper, iron, magnesium, manganese, selenium, phosphorus, potassium, zinc	asthma, arthritis, bladder disorders, blood pressure, bone problems, constipation, diabetes, fatigue, haemorrhoids, headaches, heart problems, joint problems, menopause, muscle cramps, pregnancy and childbirth, rheumatism, stress, thyroid disorders	selenium is important for cancer prevention; detoxifies liver and lowers cholesterol	use seeds without hull

A–Z of conditions with ingredients to combat them

CONDITION	FRUITS	VEGETABLES	Nuts, seeds and added extras	Suitable recipes	
acne	apple, blueberry, mango, papaya (pawpaw), strawberry	asparagus, beetroot (red beet), Brussels sprout, carrot, cucumber, green (bell) pepper, lettuce, parsnip, root ginger, spinach, turnip and turnip greens, watercress, wheatgrass	almonds, flaxseeds, pumpkin seeds, sesame seeds	Aphrodite's Love Potion Blueberry Burst Body Detox Carrot Cocktail Carrot Combat	Cucumber Cleanser Mango Tango Mr McGregor's Feast Muscle Tonic Punchy Parsnip Strawberry Fayre
anaemia	apple, apricot, banana, cherry, dates, grape, lemon, lime, orange, peach, prune	alfalfa, asparagus, beansprout, beetroot (red beet), carrots, endive, kale, lettuce, parsley, spinach, string bean, Swiss chard, tomato, turnip, watercress, wheatgrass	sesame seeds, peanuts	Body Detox Carrot Cocktail Celery Soother Cherry Aid Citrus Sensation Cucumber Cleanser	Italian Serenade Lusty Lungs Mr McGregor's Feast Muscle Tonic Orange Mint Marvel Peach Perfection Vitamin Vitality

anxiety	cantaloupe melon, grape, pineapple, strawberry	broccoli, carrot, celery, garlic, kale, parsley, red (bell) pepper, root ginger, spinach, spring greens (collard greens), Swiss chard, wheatgrass	sesame seeds, peanuts	Aloha Delight Bedtime Broccoli Garlic Guardian Melon Medley	Mr McGregor's Feast Muscle Tonic Pepper Pick-me-up Tropical Teaser
arthritis	apple, cherry, dates, goji berries, lemon, lime, nectarine, papaya (pawpaw), prune, watermelon	avocado, basil, beansprout, beetroot (red beet), carrot, courgette (zucchini), cucumber, fennel, kale, leek, parsley, parsnip, potato, radish, spinach, sweet (bell) pepper, turnip, wheatgrass	peanuts, pumpkin seeds, sesame seeds, sunflower seeds	Apple Aniseed Body Detox Carrot Cocktail Cherry Aid Cucumber Cleanser Eye Elixir Fennel Fusion Green Lite	Green Tureen Hangover Horizon Lusty Lungs Melon Medley Muscle Tonic Punchy Parsnip Vitamin Vitality
asthma	apple, banana, cranberry, lemon, lime, orange	asparagus, basil, cabbage, carrot, celery, courgette (zucchini), garlic, kale, kohlrabi, mint, parsley, parsnip, radish, red Swiss chard, spinach, spring greens (collard greens), turnip, watercress, wheatgrass	oats, sunflower seeds	Carrot Cocktail Citrus Sensation Garlic Guardian Green Lite Green Tureen Hangover Horizon Lusty Lungs	Muscle Tonic Orange Mint Marvel Peter Rabbit's Delight Punchy Parsnip Top 'n' Tail Tonic Weight Watcher's Wonder

SPECIFIC
CONDITIONS

bladder disorders	blackcurrant, blueberry, cranberry, melon, pear, plum, pomegranate, watermelon	beetroot (red beet), Brussels sprout, cabbage, carrot, courgette (zucchini), cucumber, endive, marrow, onion, parsley, parsnip, tomato, turnip, watercress, wheatgrass	almonds, flaxseeds, oats, peanuts, sunflower seeds	Blackcurrant Booster Blueberry Burst Cucumber Cleanser Hangover Horizon	Melon Medley Peter Rabbit's Delight Punchy Parsnip Purple Power
blood disorders	grape, lemon, lime, orange, papaya (pawpaw), peach, pineapple, strawberry			Aloha Delight Citrus Sensation	Hawaiian Sunrise
blood pressure problems	apricot, banana, blackberry, blueberry, dates, grape, kiwi fruit, mango, nectarine, orange, peach, pomegranate, strawberry	avocado, beetroot (red beet), Brussels sprout, cabbage, courgette (zucchini), cucumber, garlic, spinach, sweet (bell) pepper, wheatgrass	almonds, peanuts, pumpkin seeds, sesame seeds, sunflower seeds	Capital C Cardio Kiwi Green Lite Green Tureen	Orange Mint Marvel Venus Awakened Vitamin Vitality Banana Bonanza
bone problems	blackberry, dates, prunes	alfalfa, avocado, broccoli, fennel, leafy greens, parsley, parsnip, wheatgrass	almonds, peanuts, pumpkin seeds, sesame seeds, sunflower seeds, yoghurt	Apple Aniseed	Eye Elixir

condition	fruit	vegetable	recipes	
bronchitis		cabbage, celery, fennel, garlic, Swiss chard, turnip, wheatgrass	Apple Aniseed Eye Elixir	Garlic Guardian Sex Enhancer
catarrh	cherry, citrus fruit, grape, kiwi fruit	kohlrabi, radish, spring onion (scallion)	Capital C Cardio Kiwi	Cherry Aid Citrus Sensation
circulatory weakness	apple, blackberry, blackcurrant, kiwi fruit, plum, raspberry	beetroot (red beet), broccoli, cabbage, carrot, celery, cucumber, garlic, green (bell) pepper, kale, onion, parsley, potato, spinach, turnip, watercress, wheatgrass	Blackcurrant Booster Bedtime Broccoli Blueberry Burst Body Detox Capital C Cardio Kiwi Carrot Cocktail Celery Soother Cucumber Cleanser Early Energiser Garlic Guardian Green Tureen	Hearty Oats and Berries Lusty Lungs Mr McGregor's Feast Muscle Tonic Peter Rabbit's Delight Pepper Pick-me-up Purple Power Raspberry Reviver Top 'n' Tail Tonic Weight Watcher's Wonder

continued ▶

	fruits	vegetables	seeds/other	recipes
colds and flu	cranberry, goji berries, grapefruit, kiwi fruit, lemon, lime, orange, papaya (pawpaw), pineapple raspberry, strawberry	seaweed		Aloha Delight, Capital C, Cardio Kiwi, Citrus Sensation, Hawaiian Sunrise, Pineapple Paradise, Pink Nightcap, Raspberry Reviver, Venus Awakened
colitis	dates	beetroot (red beet), Brussels sprout, cabbage, cauliflower, mint, spinach, wheatgrass		Body Builder, Purple Power
constipation	apple, apricot, banana, cherry, dates, grape, lemon, lime, mango, melon, papaya (pawpaw), peach, pear, plum, pomegranate, prune, strawberry	avocado, Brussels sprout, cabbage, celery, courgette (zucchini), cucumber, endive, leek, lettuce, potato, root ginger, spinach, wheatgrass	flaxseeds, oats, pumpkin seeds, sesame seeds, sunflower seeds	Aphrodite's Love Potion, Apricot Glow, Breakfast Unblocker, Cherry Aid, Citrus Sensation, Super Commuter, Early Energiser, Ginger Digest, Green Lite, Green Tureen, Hangover Harmony, Mango Tango, Melon Medley, Peach Perfection, Peppy Papaya, Simply Apple and Pear, Strawberry Fayre, Strawberry Slumber, Vitamin Vitality, Weight Watcher's Wonder

convalescence	apple, blackcurrant, raspberry	beetroot		Blackcurrant Booster Ginger Fizz	Purple Power Raspberry Reviver
coughs	citrus fruit, kiwi fruit, papaya (pawpaw)	horseradish, mint, onion, spring onion (scallion)		Capital C Cardio Kiwi	Citrus Sensation Orange Mint Marvel
cramps	banana, cherry, papaya (pawpaw), watermelon	avocado, celery	sunflower seeds	Cherry Aid Super Commuter Hangover Harmony	Green Tureen Melon Medley Top 'n' Tail Tonic
cystitis	apple, blackcurrant, cantaloupe melon, cranberry, lemon, lime, papaya (pawpaw), pomegranate	beetroot (red beet), broccoli, carrot, celery, cucumber, green (bell) pepper, kale, parsley, spinach, spring greens (collard greens), wheatgrass		Bedtime Broccoli Blackcurrant Booster Body Detox Carrot Cocktail Citrus Sensation Early Energiser	Hangover Harmony Muscle Tonic Purple Power Top 'n' Tail Tonic Weight Watcher's Wonder
depression	banana, pineapple, raspberry	avocado, beetroot (red beet), broccoli, carrot, garlic, green (bell) pepper, kale, parsley, spinach, spring greens (collard greens), sweet potato, tomato	flaxseed, oats, walnuts, yoghurt, peanuts	Bedtime Broccoli Banana Bonanza Celery Soother Garlic Guardian	Mr McGregor's Feast Muscle Tonic Pepper Pick-me-up Raspberry Reviver

SPECIFIC
CONDITIONS

diabetes	banana, berries, green apples, orange, papaya (pawpaw)	avocado, beansprout, Brussels sprout, carrot, celery, Jerusalem artichoke, kale, lettuce, parsley, parsnip, spinach, string bean, sweet potato, tomato, turnip, wheatgrass	almonds, oats, pumpkin seeds, sesame seeds, sunflower seeds	Caribbean Calypso Celery Soother Super Commuter Firmly Rooted Hangover Horizon Mr McGregor's Feast (use green apples) Muscle Tonic	Pepper Pick-me-up Peppy Papaya Punchy Parsnip Vitamin Vitality Weight Watcher's Wonder (use green apples)
diarrhoea	apple, banana, blackberry, blueberry, cranberry, dates	beetroot (red beet), carrot, celery, parsley, potato, spinach		Carrot Cocktail Ginger Fizz Muscle Tonic	Top 'n' Tail Tonic Weight Watcher's Wonder
digestive problems	apple, banana, blackberry, cherry, grapefruit, kiwi fruit, lemon, lime, pineapple, raspberry	avocado, beansprout, Brussels sprout, cabbage, carrot, fennel, Jerusalem artichoke, onion, parsnip, potato, spinach, tomato, watercress	flaxseed, oats, sesame seeds,	Apple Aniseed Cardio Kiwi Cherry Aid Early Energiser Hawaiian Sunrise	Hearty Oats and Berries Italian Serenade Pineapple Paradise Pink Nightcap Raspberry Reviver
ear disorders	grapefruit, lemon, lime			Citrus Sensation	Pink Nightcap

eczema	apple, blackcurrants, papaya (pawpaw)	beetroot (red beet), carrot, cucumber, kohlrabi, potato, radish, root ginger, spinach, watercress		Blackcurrant Booster Body Detox Carrot Cocktail Carrot Combat Cucumber Cleanser	Lusty Lungs Muscle Tonic Peppy Papaya Purple Power
eye disorders	banana, dates, goji berries, nectarine	alfalfa, asparagus, avocado, beetroot (red beet), carrot, celery, courgette (zucchini), endive, kale, parsley, parsnip, spinach, sweet (bell) pepper, turnip, wheatgrass	pumpkin seeds, sesame seeds	Breakfast Unblocker Super Commuter Green Lite Green Tureen Mr McGregor's Feast	Muscle Tonic Pepper Pick-me-up Punchy Parsnip Venus Awakened
fatigue	banana, grapefruit, kiwi fruit, orange, pineapple, plum, raspberry	alfalfa, beans, beansprout, beetroot (red beet), broccoli, Brussels sprout, cabbage, cauliflower, celery, cucumber, garlic, Jerusalem artichoke, kale, onion, parsley, potato, red Swiss chard, root ginger, seaweed, spinach, spring greens (collard greens), turnip, wheatgrass	almonds, apple cider vinegar, oats, sunflower seeds, peanuts	Banana Bonanza Bedtime Broccoli Breakfast Unblocker Capital C Cardio Kiwi Early Energiser Firmly Rooted	Green Tureen Hawaiian Sunrise Pineapple Paradise Pink Nightcap Raspberry Reviver Tropical Teaser

continued ▶

SPECIFIC
CONDITIONS

fever	apple, apricots, citrus fruit, cranberry, grape, raspberry, strawberry	beetroot (red beet), cabbage, cucumber, garlic, onion, root ginger	Orange Mint Marvel Pink Nightcap	Raspberry Reviver Strawberry Fayre
fluid retention	cranberry, lemon, lime, strawberry, watermelon	beansprouts, celery, cucumber, fenugreek	Early Energiser Hangover Harmony	Melon Medley
gallstones	cherry, increased intake of fruit and vegetables	increased intake of fruit and vegetables	Cherry Aid	
gout	apple, cherry, citrus fruit, grape, papaya (pawpaw), pineapple, strawberry	asparagus, carrot, celery, fennel, parsley, spinach, string bean, tomato	Aloha Delight Aphrodite's Love Potion Apple Aniseed Celery Soother Cherry Aid Carrot Cocktail Early Energiser Eye Elixir Hangover Horizon Italian Serenade	Muscle Tonic Mr McGregor's Feast Orange Mint Marvel Peppy Papaya Pink Nightcap Sex Enhancer Strawberry Fayre Top 'n' Tail Tonic Weight Watcher's Wonder

	fruits	vegetables	other	recipes	
haemorrhoids	apple, grape, prune	carrot, potato, spinach, turnip, watercress	flaxseeds, oats, sunflower seeds, walnuts	Carrot Cocktail Lusty Lungs	Muscle Tonic
hair loss	lime	alfalfa, cabbage, carrot, cucumber, kale, lettuce, spinach, sweet (bell) pepper, watercress, wheatgrass	flaxseeds, Greek yoghurt, sesame seeds, walnuts	Citrus Sensation Cucumber Cleanser	Mr McGregor's Feast Pepper Pick-me-up
halitosis	citrus fruit	cabbage, carrot, cucumber, mint, root ginger, spinach		Carrot Combat Citrus Sensation Muscle Tonic	Orange Mint Marvel Peter Rabbit's Delight
hangover	cherry, citrus fruit, grapefruit, mango, pineapple, melon	avocado, beetroot (red beet), broccoli, cabbage, carrot, cauliflower, celery, cucumber, kale, root ginger, tomato	walnuts	Aphrodite's Love Potion Body Detox Caribbean Calypso Carrot Combat Cherry Aid Hangover Harmony	Hangover Horizon Hawaiian Sunrise Melon Medley Pineapple Paradise Pink Nightcap Tropical Teaser
hay fever	grapefruit, orange, strawberry	kale, parsnip, wheatgrass		Capital C Hawaiian Sunrise	Punchy Parsnip (omit apple)

continued ▶

SPECIFIC
CONDITIONS

	fruits	vegetables	nuts/seeds	recipes	recipes
headache and migraine	apple, cantaloupe melon	avocado, celery, fennel, garlic, parsley, root ginger, spring greens (collard greens)	almonds, pumpkin seeds, sunflower seeds	Apple Aniseed, Celery Soother, Ginger Digest, Melon Medley	Sex Enhancer, Weight Watcher's Wonder
heart problems	banana, blackberry, blackcurrant, dates, goji berries, kiwi, nectarine, orange, papaya (pawpaw)	avocado, beetroot (red beet), Brussels sprout, courgette (zucchini), endive, fenugreek, Jerusalem artichoke, parsley, spinach, spring onion (scallion), sweet (bell) pepper, turnip, wheatgrass	almonds, oats, pumpkin seeds, sesame seeds, sunflower seeds, peanuts	Blackcurrant Booster, Breakfast Unbloker, Capital C, Super Commuter, Green Lite, Green Tureen	Hearty Oats and Berries, Muscle Tonic, Purple Power, Vitamin Vitality
impotence	berries, cherry, dates	alfalfa, beetroot (red beet), kale, wheatgrass	soya milk, tofu	Cherry Aid, Cucumber Cleanser	Purple Power
indigestion	apple, banana, cherry, citrus fruit, grape, mango, melon, papaya (pawpaw), peach, pineapple, strawberry	asparagus, broccoli, carrot, cauliflower, celery, mint, potato, root ginger	oats, sesame seeds	Bedtime Broccoli, Cherry Aid, Peppy Papaya, Aphrodite's Love Potion, Carrot Cocktail, Carrot Combat, Citrus Sensation	Early Energiser, Mango Tango, Melon Medley, Orange Mint Marvel, Peach Perfection, Top 'n' Tail Tonic, Weight Watcher's Wonder

infection	lemon, lime	Brussels sprout, seaweed, spinach, turnip, wheatgrass	oats		Citrus Sensation
insomnia	banana, blueberries, grapefruit, lime, pear	broccoli, carrots, celery, lettuce, parsley	peanuts, pumpkin seeds, sesame seeds	Bedtime Broccoli, Banana Bonanza, Citrus Sensation	Simply Apple and Pear, Strawberry Slumber, Pink Nightcap
joint problems	apple, berries, cherry	basil, broccoli, garlic, leek	almonds, flaxseeds, pumpkin seeds, sesame seeds, sunflower seeds, walnuts, peanuts	Bedtime Broccoli, Blueberry Burst, Blackcurrant Booster	Cherry Aid, Italian Serenade
kidney disorders — must watch potassium levels	apple, blueberry, cranberry, goji berries, grape, lemon, lime, mango, melon, papaya (pawpaw), pineapple, strawberry	alfalfa, asparagus, avocado, beetroot (red beet), cabbage, carrot, cauliflower, celery, cucumber, fennel, parsley, spinach, sweet (bell) pepper, tomato, turnip, watercress, wheatgrass		Aloha Delight, Aphrodite's Love Potion, Apple Aniseed, Caribbean Calypso, Celery Soother, Early Energiser, Fennel Fusion, Hangover Harmony	Mango Tango, Muscle Tonic, Peppy Papaya, Sex Enhancer, Strawberry Fayre, Tropical Teaser, Weight Watcher's Wonder, Vitamin Vitality

continued ▶

	fruits	vegetables	seeds/nuts	recipes
laryngitis		beetroot (red beet), carrot, cucumber, spinach		Purple Power
liver disorders	apple, berries, citrus fruits, goji berries, grape, grapefruit, kiwi, mango, orange, papaya (pawpaw), pear	alfalfa, asparagus, avocado, beans, Brussels sprouts, beetroot (red beet), cabbage, carrot, cauliflower, celery, cucumber, endive, fennel, garlic, Jerusalem artichoke, kale, lettuce, parsley, parsnip, spinach, tomato, turnip, watercress, wheatgrass	pumpkin seeds, sesame seeds, walnuts	Body Detox, Cucumber Cleanser, Apple Aniseed, Capital C, Carrot Cocktail, Celery Soother, Citrus Sensation, Cucumber Cleanser, Early Energiser, Eye Elixir, Fennel Fusion, Garlic Guardian, Green Tureen, Ginger Digest, Hangover Horizon, Italian Serenade, Lusty Lungs, Mango Tango, Mr McGregor's Feast, Muscle Tonic, Orange Mint Marvel, Pepper Pick-me-up, Peppy Papaya, Peter Rabbit's Delight, Pink Nightcap, Carrot Cocktail, Carrot Combat, Hangover Horizon, Lusty Lungs, Muscle Tonic, Orange Mint Marvel, Punchy Parsnip, Purple Power, Sex Enhancer, Simply Apple and Pear, Top 'n' Tail Tonic, Weight Watcher's Wonder

	fruits	vegetables	nuts/seeds	recipes	
lung disorders	apple, cranberry, dates, orange	carrot, kohlrabi, parsley, potato, radish, root ginger, turnip, watercress		Carrot Cocktail Carrot Combat Hangover Horizon	Lusty Lungs Muscle Tonic Orange Mint Marvel
menopause	apple, blackberry, blackcurrant, blueberry, dates, grapefruit, orange, pear, pineapple, pomegranate, strawberry	beetroot (red beet), carrot, celery, parsley, spinach, Swiss chard, tomato	flaxseeds, maca powder, nuts, oats, pumpkin seeds, sesame seeds, sunflower seeds, peanuts	Aloha Delight Aphrodite's Love Potion Blackcurrant Booster Breakfast Unblocker Carrot Cocktail Celery Soother Early Energiser Ginger Digest Hangover Horizon Hawaiian Sunrise Hearty Oats and Berries	Italian Serenade Mr McGregor's feast Muscle Tonic Orange Mint Marvel Pineapple Paradise Pink Nightcap Purple Power Simply Apple and Pear Strawberry Fayre Strawberry Slumber Top 'n' Tail Tonic Weight Watcher's Wonder

continued ▶

SPECIFIC
CONDITIONS

SPECIFIC CONDITIONS

menstrual problems	apple, banana, cherry, grape, pineapple	beetroot (red beet), fennel, Swiss chard, watercress		Aloha Delight Apple Aniseed Cherry Aid	Cucumber Cleanser Fennel Fusion Strawberry Slumber
motion sickness	berries, strawberry	broccoli, kale, lettuce, mint, root ginger, spinach, sweet (bell) pepper, turnip greens		Blackcurrant Booster Mr McGregor's Feast	Strawberry Fayre
mouth ulcers	cantaloupe melon, cranberry	cabbage, carrot, celery, root ginger, spinach, spring greens (collard greens), wheatgrass		Carrot Combat Melon Medley	Peter Rabbit's Delight
muscular problems	banana, pineapple	asparagus, beansprout, beetroot (red beet), carrot, celery, courgette (zucchini), cucumber, kale, lettuce, parsley, parsnip, potato, red (bell) pepper, spinach, spring greens (collard greens), Swiss chard, watercress	sunflower seeds	Celery Soother Cucumber Cleanser Early Energiser Green Lite	Green Tureen Lusty Lungs Mr McGregor's Feast Muscle Tonic

nausea	apple, banana, lemon, lime, strawberry	broccoli, kale, lettuce, root ginger, spinach, sweet (bell) pepper, turnip greens		Citrus Sensation	Strawberry Fayre
nervous disorders	lime, raspberry	asparagus, beetroot (red beet), Brussels sprout, carrot, celery, fennel, lettuce, spinach, wheatgrass		Body Detox Eye Elixir Fennel Fusion	Raspberry Reviver Sex Enhancer
pneumonia	lemon, lime, orange, pineapple, strawberry			Aloha Delight Aphrodite's Love Potion	Citrus Sensation
pregnancy and childbirth	banana, blackberry, dates, grapefruit, peach, pineapple	alfalfa, courgette (zucchini), kale, root ginger, parsnip	almonds, pumpkin seeds, sunflower seeds, walnuts	Breakfast Unblocker Early Energiser Hawaiian Sunrise	Pineapple Paradise Tropical Teaser
prostate disorders	apple, cherry, cranberry, dates, pear, pomegranate, strawberry, watermelon	asparagus, beetroot (red beet), carrot, celery, courgette (zucchini), cucumber, lettuce, root ginger, parsley, spinach, tomato	pumpkin seeds	Body Detox Carrot Cocktail Carrot Combat Cherry Aid Celery Soother	Cucumber Cleanser Ginger Digest Green Lite Hangover Harmony

continued ▶

respiratory problems	apple, dates, blackcurrant	carrot, garlic, leek, onion, root ginger, watercress	sesame seeds	Blackcurrant Booster Carrot Cocktail Carrot Combat Lusty Lungs Purple Power Italian Serenade Melon Medley	Muscle Tonic Simply Apple and Pear Strawberry Fayre Top 'n' Tail Tonic Weight Watcher's Wonder
rheumatism	apple, cherry, grape, lemon, lime, orange, strawberry	asparagus, beans, beetroot (red beet), carrot, celery, cucumber, watercress	almonds, peanuts, sunflower seeds	Body Detox Carrot Cocktail Cherry Aid Citrus Sensation Cucumber Cleanser Early Energiser	Hangover Horizon Orange Mint Marvel Strawberry Fayre Top 'n' Tail Tonic Weight Watcher's Wonder
sciatica	apple, apricot, berries, cherry, mango, papaya (pawpaw), pineapple	broccoli, carrot, leafy greens, spinach, sweet (bell) pepper, tomato	almonds, flaxseeds, peanuts, walnuts	Apricot Glow Bedtime Broccoli Blackcurrant Booster Caribbean Calypso Carrot Cocktail Cherry Aid Italian Serenade	Mango Tango Mr McGregor's Feast Muscle Tonic Pepper Pick-me-up Peppy Papaya Vitamin Vitality

				Carrot Combat	Punchy Parsnip
sinusitis	mango, papaya (pawpaw)	alfalfa, carrot, garlic, kohlrabi, parsnip, radish, root ginger, tomato			
skin disorders	apricot, blackberry, citrus fruit, cranberry, goji berries, grape, kiwi fruit, nectarine, watermelon	asparagus, beetroot (red beet), cabbage, carrot, cucumber, endive, fennel, fenugreek, garlic, kale, kohlrabi, parsley, parsnip, radish, spinach, spring onion (scallion), string bean, sweet (bell) pepper, Swiss chard, tomato, turnip, watercress, wheatgrass	pumpkin seeds	Apricot Glow Body Detox Capital C Cardio Kiwi Cucumber Cleanser Eye Elixir Fennel Fusion Garlic Guardian	Hangover Harmony Mr McGregor's Feast Muscle Tonic Orange Mint Marvel Pepper Pick-me-up Peter Rabbit's Delight Punchy Parsnip Purple Power
sore throat	blackcurrant, citrus fruit, kiwi fruit, papaya (pawpaw), pineapple, pomegranate	root ginger		Blackcurrant Booster Capital C Cardio Kiwi Citrus Sensation	Hawaiian Sunrise Pineapple Paradise Tropical Teaser

continued ▶

SPECIFIC CONDITIONS

	Fruits	Vegetables	Nuts and seeds	Recipes	
stress	banana, cantaloupe melon, grape, kiwi fruit, pineapple, strawberry	broccoli, cabbage, carrot, celery, garlic, kale, parsley, red (bell) pepper, root ginger, spinach, spring greens (collard greens), Swiss chard, tomato, wheatgrass	peanuts, pumpkin seeds, sesame seeds, sunflower seeds	Aloha Delight, Aphrodite's Love Potion, Bedtime Broccoli, Banana Bonanza, Capital C, Cardio Kiwi, Carrot Combat	Celery Soother, Garlic Guardian, Melon Medley, Mr McGregor's Feast, Muscle Tonic, Pepper Pick-me-up, Strawberry Slumber, Tropical Teaser
thrush		avocado, beetroot (red beet), baby marrow, broccoli, cabbage, carrot, cauliflower, celery, cucumber, garlic, kale, leafy greens, lettuce, parsley, radish, red Swiss chard, root ginger, seaweed, spinach, sweet (bell) pepper, tomato, turnip greens		Celery Soother, Cucumber Cleanser, Early Energiser, Garlic Guardian	Green Tureen, Mr McGregor's Feast, Muscle Tonic, Pepper Pick-me-up
thyroid disorders	blueberry, raspberry, strawberry	alfalfa, kohlrabi, radish, seaweed, spinach, sweet (bell) pepper, watercress	Brazil nuts, chia seeds, oat bran, sunflower seeds	Raspberry Reviver, Strawberry Fayre	Venus Awakened
ulcers	banana, cranberry, mango, papaya (pawpaw)	cabbage, carrot, kale, parsnip, potato, spinach, wheatgrass		Mango Tango, Muscle Tonic	Peter Rabbit's Delight, Punchy Parsnip

Condition				Juices & smoothies
urinary tract disorders	blackcurrant, blueberry, cherry, cranberry	beetroot (red beet), garlic, leek, parsley, sweet (bell) pepper, tomato, watercress		Blackcurrant Booster, Blueberry Burst, Cherry Aid, Cucumber Cleanser, Pepper Pick-me-up, Purple Power
varicose veins	blueberry, grapefruit, lemon, orange, watermelon	asparagus, broccoli, carrot, potato, root ginger, spinach, tomato, turnip, watercress		Blueberry Burst, Cucumber Cleanser, Hangover Harmony, Lusty Lungs, Melon Medley, Muscle Tonic, Pink Nightcap
weight loss (obesity)	apple, cherry, citrus fruit, cranberry, dates, goji berries, grape, kiwi fruit, mango, nectarine, papaya (pawpaw), pineapple, prune, strawberry, watermelon	alfalfa, avocado, beansprout, beetroot (red beet), carrot, celery, courgette (zucchini), cucumber, endive, fennel, fenugreek, Jerusalem artichoke, kale, kohlrabi, lettuce, parsley, parsnip, seaweed, spinach, spring onion (scallion), tomato, turnip, watercress, wheatgrass	almonds, flaxseeds	All those in chapter 3 plus: Apple Aniseed, Body Detox, Capital C, Cardio Kiwi, Caribbean Calypso, Carrot Cocktail, Celery Soother, Cherry Aid, Citrus Sensation, Cucumber Cleanser, Early Energiser, Eye Elixir, Green Tureen, Hangover Harmony, Hangover Horizon, Mango Tango, Mr McGregor's Feast, Muscle Tonic, Orange Mint Marvel, Peter Rabbit's Delight, Punchy Parsnip, Sex Enhancer, Strawberry Fayre, Venus Awakened, Vitamin Vitality

Appendix 1
Vitamins and minerals

Vitamins

There are 13 essential vitamins that facilitate the metabolic processes of the body, for example, the metabolism of carbohydrates, fats and proteins to produce energy, the building up of the body proteins, the absorption of calcium for the gut and bones, the multiplication of body cells, and the formation of blood cells. Without their presence we simply could not exist.

VITAMIN A (RETINOL)

Fat soluble. The vision vitamin, the deficiency of which has a marked effect on the eyes that can lead to blindness or xerophthalmia. Vitamin A is found in animal foods or as carotenoids (which gives carrots their colour) in some vegetables and fruit. Carotenoids, which can be converted by the body into vitamin A, protect against cancers, in particular those on surface tissues, inside the lungs, and of the breast, intestines, stomach, bladder and skin. Vitamin A taken in excess in tablet form can be poisonous to the liver and cause damage; B-carotene taken in excess can cause a temporary orange colour to the skin, which is not harmful.

Sources
Apricots, butter, broccoli, carrots, cheese, cod liver oil, eggs, fish oils, fortified margarines, kale, kidney, liver, mango, melon, milk, oranges, papaya (pawpaw), peaches, peas, peppers, pumpkin, spinach, sweet potato, squash, tomatoes, wheatgrass

VITAMIN B1 (THIAMINE)

Water soluble. Helps maintain the nervous system and plays an essential role in carbohydrate metabolism. Wholegrains are typically rich in thiamine content but most is removed during processing. It is also easily destroyed by heat, so cooking losses are high.

Sources
Beans, beansprouts, fortified cereal foods, cod's roe, duck, fruit, milk, nuts, oatmeal, peas, pork, potatoes, vegetables such as alfalfa sprouts, wheatgerm, wholemeal bread and flour, yeast and yeast extract

VITAMIN B2 (RIBOFLAVIN)

Water soluble. For healthy skin, eyes, hair and growth in general. It is essential to carbohydrate, amino acid and fat metabolism and provides antioxidant protection.

Sources
Bananas, bread, broccoli, cereals, cheese, chicken, cottage cheese, eggs, fish, fortified breakfast cereals, green vegetables, kelp, liver, meat, milk, mushrooms, nuts, spinach, sprouted beans and grains, wheat bran, wheatgerm, yeast, yoghurt

VITAMIN B3 (NIACIN)

Water soluble. Like thiamine and riboflavin, niacin is involved in the process by which energy is released from the cells within the body.

Sources
Much the same as riboflavin foods – beans, bran, brewer's yeast, coffee, fish, fortified breakfast cereals, kelp, kidney, lean meat, liver, milk, mushrooms, peanuts, peas, pine nuts, rice, sesame seeds, sprouted beans and grains, sunflower seeds, tomatoes, vegetables, wholemeal bread and flour, yeast extract

VITAMIN B5 (PANTOTHENIC ACID)

Water soluble. Like thiamine and riboflavin, and niacin, it is involved in the process by which energy is released from the cells within the body and for healthy skin. Pantothenic acid is essential for growth. Pantothenic acid also plays a role in the production of hormones and cholesterol.

Sources
Small quantities of pantothenic acid are found in most foods. Avocados, beans, broccoli, cabbage, chicken organ meats, eggs, kale, lentils, meats, milk, mushrooms, potatoes, sweet potato, wholegrains

VITAMIN B6 (PYRIDOXINE)
Water soluble. Involved in the metabolism of amino acids and necessary to help make up the haemoglobin in blood. Vitamin B6 is needed for the biosynthesis of the neurotransmitters serotonin. It is claimed that extra B6 can help relieve depression caused by the contraceptive pill and premenstrual tension.

Sources
Avocados, bananas, beans, bread, chicken, meats, nuts and seeds, tuna, vegetables, wholegrains, yeast extract

VITAMIN B12 (COBALAMIN)
Water soluble. A mixture of several related compounds and needed for rapidly dividing cells such as those in the digestive tract, nervous tissue and bone marrow from which blood is formed. As it is found in animal foods it is customary for vegans to obtain their supply from plant 'milks' such as soya milk or yeast extracts that have been fortified with B12.

Sources
Cheese, eggs, fortified cereals, heart, kidney, liver, meat, milk, oily fish, oysters, seaweed, wheatgrass, yoghurt

FOLATE
Needed for rapidly dividing cells such as blood cells. An increased intake is necessary during pregnancy. Periconceptual folate supplementation can reduce the risk of birth defects and neural tube defects. Folate is easily destroyed during cooking.

Asparagus, avocados, bananas, beetroot (red beet), bran, broccoli, butter (lima) beans, cabbage, Chinese leaf (stem lettuce), eggs, some fish, fortified cereals, kidney, lettuce, liver, mushrooms, meats, oranges, peanuts, raw leafy green vegetables, spinach, wholemeal bread

VITAMIN C (ASCORBIC ACID)

Water soluble. Vitamin C has a number of useful functions. It helps keep the structure of connective tissue healthy, and it enables iron to be more easily absorbed. It also aids recovery from illness and contributes to healthy bones, teeth, gums and blood vessels and inhibits a group of cancer-causing agents. It is recommended to be increased by patients undergoing surgery, as it plays an important part in healing wounds and connective tissue (some hospitals advise patients to increase their daily dose by almost ten times by taking 1 litre/1¾ pt of orange juice a few days before the operation). An increase is also helpful for drug takers and smokers. Scientists have confirmed that overdosing is harmful and can cause excess amounts of oxalate (a calcium compound) in the urine, which can form stones in the bladder. Tablet overdosing can be harmful and the best course is to eat more fruit and vegetables, thereby getting the benefit of other vitamins and minerals. Potatoes are not a concentrated form of vitamin C, but because they are eaten in large quantities, they contribute a useful amount.

Sources
Blackcurrants, blueberries, broccoli, Brussels sprouts, lightly cooked cabbage, cauliflower, citrus fruit (grapefruit, lemons, limes, orange), guavas, kiwi fruit, pineapple, potatoes, rosehip syrup, strawberries, sweet (bell) peppers (all colours), tomatoes, wheatgrass

VITAMIN D (CALCIFEROL)

Fat soluble. Vitamin D is known as the sunshine vitamin as it is made in the skin on modest exposure to sunlight. Because it can be made in the body, has specific target tissues and does not have to be supplied in the diet, it can be considered a hormone. It is needed in the regulation of more than 50 genes in the body. Vitamin D helps to regulate calcium and phosphorus

SPECIFIC CONDITIONS

levels in the bones and teeth. A level of calcium is essential for the action of muscles like the heart and to help the nerves to function properly. It is very easy to overdose in the tablet form, which can cause hypercalcaemia – too much calcium in the soft tissue – resulting in thirst, loss of appetite, headaches, nausea and vomiting.

Sources
Butter, cod liver oil, eggs, fatty fish, fish liver oils, fortified breakfast cereals, fortified margarines, fortified milk and milk substitutes, herring, liver, mackerel, pilchards, salmon, sardines, sunlight, tuna

VITAMIN E (TOCOPHEROL)

Fat soluble. Vitamin E is a strong antioxidant: it protects essential fatty acids from the destructive effects of oxygen. It is a natural anti-coagulant, aids reproduction, promotes healthy skin, and its antioxidant powers protect against heart disease and cancer.

Sources
Avocado, beetroot (red beet), broccoli, butter, carrots, celery, eggs, fortified cereals, leafy green vegetables, margarine, milk, nuts and seeds, olive oil, olives, spinach, sprouted grains, sunflower seeds, tomatoes, vegetable oils, wheatgerm, wheatgrass, wholegrain cereals

VITAMIN K (NAPTHAQUINONE)

Fat soluble. Found mainly in vegetables but also produced by bacteria in the gut. An essential vitamin for the normal clotting of the blood, it plays a role in bone formation, and helps regulate numerous enzyme systems in the body. Vitamin K plays a role in age-related bone loss, heart health and regulation of inflammation in the body.

Sources
Alfalfa, asparagus, broccoli, Brussels sprouts, cabbage, carrot tops, cauliflower, chickpeas, dark green vegetables, eggs, grains, green tea, kale, kelp, lentils, lettuce (dark green), liver, meat, milk, pork, soya oil, sprouted grains, strawberries, turnip greens

Minerals

Research into minerals essential to humans is making rapid advances and scientific knowledge is constantly changing.

Minerals cannot be dissolved in water, so they are difficult to absorb and not easily excreted, except sodium, potassium, chloride, iodide and fluoride which are easily absorbed. However, our bodies do not usually suffer deficiencies, except for iron. Excessive sweating can cause cramping from loss of sodium. Most minerals in the body are found in the bones. Minerals give bones their strength and hardness; without them they would be like rubber. Minerals represent 4 to 5 per cent of our body weight. The most common mineral in the bones is calcium, which accounts for 50 per cent of this weight but phosphorous is also important and small amounts of magnesium.

CALCIUM

Needed daily. Calcium is the most abundant mineral in the body; it makes up 1.5 to 2 per cent of our total body weight and accounts for 39 per cent of our total body minerals. Approximately 50 per cent of the calcium in food is passed out of the body, so the recommended intakes are about three times higher than the amount actually needed. Approximately 99 per cent of the remaining calcium is transported to the skeleton by vitamin D and the remaining 1 per cent performs the vitally important function of triggering muscle contractions, including those of the heart muscles, and nerve function, for the activity of several enzymes, and for normal clotting of the blood. Ageing, crash diets, high salt intake, and chronic gastrointestinal diseases lead to calcium loss, and high consumption of alcohol, coffee, meat, bran, salt and cola drinks make it more difficult for calcium to be absorbed. In the UK, all bread except wholemeal is fortified with extra calcium. Calcium absorption is enhanced if calcium is taken as part of a meal. Higher calcium intakes are associated with a decreased prevalence of being overweight and obese.

Sources

Bread and flour, cheese, canned fish (where the bones are eaten), dried figs, dulse, fortified cereals, green vegetables, hard water, kelp, milk and milk products, fortified milk substitutes, nuts, parsley, peanuts, spinach, tofu, wheatgrass, yoghurt

CHROMIUM

Chromium is defined as a nutrient. It is part of the glucose tolerance factor, which enhances the action of insulin in carbohydrate metabolism and influences protein and fat metabolism. Chromium also regulates gene expression and in combination with vitamin C and vitamin E minimises oxidative stress within the body.

Sources

Apples, bananas, bran, Brewer's yeast, broccoli, cheese, chicken, garlic, grapes, green beans, liver, meats, oranges, oysters, potatoes, seafood, wholegrains

COBALT

Most of the cobalt in the body exists with vitamin B12 stores in the liver. Only one enzyme has an established specific requirement for cobalt.

COPPER

Copper is a normal component of blood. Copper works with iron in the formation of haemoglobin and occurs in melanin pigments in skin and hair. Copper is also a component of many enzymes in the body.

Sources

Found in a wide variety of food. Animal products, except milk; liver, organ meats, shellfish; also useful amounts in bread, beans, cereals, dried fruit, lentils, meat and vegetables

FLUORIDE

Found in bones and teeth. Fluoride adds considerably to the strength of tooth enamel. Adults often obtain 1 mg of fluoride from tea alone each day.

Sources

Fluoride in mains water supplies, fish, seafood: clams, oysters, sardines, and other saltwater fish, tea

IODINE

Iodine is essential in the thyroid gland, where it is a component of the hormones produced there. Unlike other minerals, iodine is easily absorbed. It is sometimes given to those who are exposed to large doses of radiation.

Warning: do not use any iodine products available from chemists' shelves on your food.

Sources
Cereals, dulse, fortified salt, kelp, seafood, vegetables

IRON

Approximately 70 per cent of iron in the body is found in haemoglobin in the blood, the other half in muscle tissue. Iron, therefore, is necessary for the production of red blood cells. Haemoglobin is essential for transferring oxygen in your blood from the lungs to the tissues. Myoglobin, in muscle cells, accepts, stores, transports and releases oxygen. A shortage of iron results in anaemia. An adequate intake of iron is essential for the normal functioning of the immune system and cognitive function. When anaemia is diagnosed a diet containing plenty of iron and vitamin C, which enhances iron absorption, should be sufficient remedy. Tea hinders iron absorption, so do not drink tea until one hour after an iron-rich meal or drink.

Sources
Dried apricots, beans, fortified cereals, chocolate, curry powder, dried fruit, dulse, egg yolks, fish, kelp, lentils, liver, nuts and seeds, potatoes, red meat, red wine, soya, soy sauce, tofu, vegetables

MAGNESIUM

Magnesium is also found in the bones (60 per cent), the muscles (26 per cent) and the remainder in the soft tissue and body fluids. It is absolutely necessary for every biochemical process in our bodies, including neuromuscular transmission and activity, in learning and memory, metabolism and the synthesis of both nucleic acids and proteins. Magnesium deficiency has been detected in people with migraine headaches, severe asthma, leg

SPECIFIC CONDITIONS

cramps, diabetes, chronic renal failure, osteoporosis, and heart and vascular disease. Diets high in protein, alcohol, vitamin D and calcium increase the requirements for magnesium.

Sources
Widespread in foods, particularly apples, bananas, brown rice, fish, leafy green vegetables, meat, milk, oranges, nuts, seeds, tofu, vegetables, wholegrain cereals, wholemeal bread

MANGANESE

Manganese is associated with the formation of connective tissue, growth and reproduction. It is essential for proper metabolism of amino acids, proteins and lipids. A deficiency can cause slow hair growth and poor pancreatic function. It also affects reproduction and aspects of carbohydrate metabolism.

Sources
Beans, coffee, leafy green vegetables, nuts, spices, tea, wholegrain cereals

PHOSPHORUS

Phosphorus is found mainly in the bones and teeth. It works with calcium, but some is needed for a chemical reaction that releases energy from the cells within the body. It is more widely distributed in food than calcium. A deficiency is virtually impossible except for someone with renal disease who is taking phosphate binders, or the elderly, whose intake may be poor.

Sources
Baking powder, beans, carrots, cheese spreads, dark green vegetables, dulse, eggs, fish, kelp, lentils, meat and meat products, milk and milk products, nuts, potatoes, tofu, wholegrain cereal products, wholemeal bread

POTASSIUM

Potassium is an electrolyte with a number of important functions in our bodies. It is important in nerve and muscle function, helps to regulate heart rhythm, regulates fluid balance and helps bones retain calcium. It is also vital in maintaining normal blood pressure as it counters the effects of sodium, which raises blood pressure. Getting the right balance of these two vitamins is vital to good heart health. Healthy kidneys keep blood potassium within a normal range but those with kidney disease, diabetes or heart failure are at risk of potassium overload as they may not be able to efficiently eliminate any excess. This may also be true for those taking certain medications for high blood pressure and heart disease.

Sources

Present in most fruit and vegetables; higher levels in avocados, bananas, beetroot, blackcurrants, broccoli, Brussels sprouts, cauliflower, celery, courgettes, fennel, garlic, ginger, goji berries, kale, kiwis, Jerusalem artichokes, parsley, parsnips, plums, potato, prunes, seaweed, spinach, squash, sweet potato, tomatoes and watercress. Also found in almonds, cheese, eggs, fish, meat, milk, sunflower seeds, wholemeal bread and yoghurt.

SELENIUM

Like vitamin E, selenium helps to prevent oxidation of essential fatty acids but, unlike vitamin E, selenium can be toxic in high concentration.

Sources

Fish, meats, milk, nuts, organ meats, oysters, seeds, wheatgerm, wholegrain cereals, wholemeal bread

ZINC

Zinc is found in cells throughout the body. It is needed for the body's immune system to properly work. Zinc plays important roles in cell division, cell growth, wound healing, and in the breakdown of carbohydrates. Zinc is also needed for the senses of smell and taste. During pregnancy, infancy and childhood the body needs zinc to grow and develop properly. It is found in the highest concentrations in the liver, pancreas, kidneys, bones and muscles but also in the eyes, prostate, skin and hair. A lack of zinc can result in hair loss and boils and swelling all over the skin.

Sources

Fish, fortified cereals, meat, milk and milk products

Appendix 2 Nutritional content of fruits and vegetables

The following data has been taken from McCance and Widdowson's *The Composition of Foods 7*th edition, produced by Food Databank National Capability in collaboration with British Nutrition Foundation, the Royal Society of Chemistry and two analytical laboratories (Eurofins and LGC). It contains nutritional information on almost 1,200 items, providing the most recent data on the foods currently eaten in the UK diet.

The charts show the composition of whole raw fruits and vegetables weighing 100 g/4 oz before being juiced. Don't be daunted by such lists of figures. For the most interesting reading, follow the line indicated for each item; for instance, on the vitamin pages find the amount of beta-carotene (vitamin A) that is given for carrots, spinach, the outer leaves of cabbages and lettuces, and compare the figures with that for pink and white grapefruit and apricots, blood oranges, cantaloupe melons, mangos and turnip tops (all cancer-fighting fruits and vegetables). Also, on the mineral pages, note the amount of minerals that can be found in 100 g/4 oz of parsley and watercress, and the potassium in prunes!

* N indicates that a nutrient is present in significant quantities but there is no reliable information on the amount.

* Tr indicates trace.

* Figures in brackets indicate an estimated value.

Vitamins

Data relates to quantities per 100 g/4 oz of whole raw fruits or vegetables before being juiced.

Food	Carotene g	Vit D g	Vit E mg	Thiamin mg	Riboflavin mg	Niacin mg	Tryptophan mg	Vit B6 mg	Vit B12 g	Folate g	Pantothenate mg	Biotin g	Vit C mg
Alfalfa sprouts	96	0	N	0.04	0.06	0.5	0.6	0.03	0	36	0.56	N	2
Almonds, flaked and ground	0	0	23.96	0.21	0.75	3.1	3.4	0.15	0	48	0.44	64	0
Apples, cooking, peeled (Unpeeled cooking apples contain 20 mg vitamin C per 100 g/4 oz.)	Tr	0	0.12	0.04	0.02	0.1	0.1	0.06	0	5	Tr	1.2	14
Apples, eating, average	14	0	0.09	0.04	0.04	0.1	Tr	0.07	0	Tr	0.10	1.1	6
Apples, Cox's Pippin	(18)	0	0.59	0.03	0.03	0.2	0.1	0.08	0	4	Tr	1.2	9
Apples, Golden Delicious	15	0	0.59	0.03	0.03	0.1	0.1	0.11	0	1	Tr	1.2	4
Apples, Granny Smith	5	0	0.59	0.04	0.02	0.1	0.1	0.08	0	1	Tr	1.2	4
Apples, red dessert (Storage may considerably affect vitamin C levels in all apples.)	15	0	0.59	0.03	0.02	0.1	0.1	0.04		1	Tr	1.2	3

continued ▶

133

Food	Carotene g	Vit D g	Vit E mg	Thiamin mg	Riboflavin mg	Niacin mg	Tryptophan mg	Vit B6 mg	Vit B12 g	Folate g	Pantothenate mg	Biotin g	Vit C mg
Apricots	405	0	N	0.04	0.05	0.5	0.1	0.08	0	5	0.24	N	6
Artichoke, Jerusalem (boiled in unsalted water)	20	0.0	0.20	0.10	Tr	0.9	0.4	N	0	N	N	N	2
Asparagus	315	0	1.16	0.16	0.06	1.0	0.5	0.09	0	175	0.17	(0.4)	12
Avocado (average, flesh only)	16	0	3.20	0.10	0.18	1.1	0.3	0.36	0.0	11	1.10	3.6	6
Banana, raw	26	0	0.16	0.15	0.04	0.7	0.2	0.31	0.0	14	0.35	2.5	9
Basil, fresh	3950	0	N	0.08	0.31	1.1	N	N	0.0	N	N	N	26
Beans, green or French	(330)	0	0.20	0.05	0.07	0.9	0.5	0.05	0	(80)	0.09	1.0	12
Beansprouts, mung	40	0	N	0.11	0.04	0.5	0.5	0.10	0	61	0.38	N	7
Beetroot (red beet)	20	0	Tr	0.01	0.01	0.1	0.3	0.03	0	150	0.12	Tr	5
Blackberries	80	0	2.37	0.02	0.05	0.5	0.1	0.05	0	34	0.25	0.4	15
Blackcurrants (Levels of vitamin C in blackcurrants ranged from 150 to 230 mg per 100 g/4 oz.)	100	0	1.00	0.03	0.06	0.3	0.1	0.08	0	N	0.40	2.4	200
Blueberries	14	0.0	0.94	0.04	0.04	0.3	0.2	0.01	0.0	8	0.20	1.5	6
Broccoli, green	575	0	(1.30)	0.10	0.06	0.9	0.8	0.14	0	90	N	N	87
Brussels sprouts	215	0	1.00	0.15	0.11	0.2	0.7	0.37	0	135	1.00	0.4	115

Food	Carotene g	Vit D g	Vit E mg	Thiamin mg	Riboflavin mg	Niacin mg	Tryptophan mg	Vit B6 mg	Vit B12 g	Folate g	Pantothenate mg	Biotin g	Vit C mg
Cabbage, average	227	0	0.06	0.28	0.03	0.5	0.2	0.13	0	65	0.28	0.1	48
Cabbage, Chinese	70	0	N	0.09	Tr	0.2	0.2	0.11	0	77	0.11	Tr	21
Cabbage, January King	340	0	0.20	0.22	0.02	0.3	0.3	0.22	0	78	0.21	0.1	49
Cabbage, red	15	0	0.20	0.02	0.01	0.4	0.2	0.09	0	39	0.32	0.1	55
Cabbage, Savoy	995	0	0.20	0.15	0.03	0.7	0.3	0.19	0	150	0.21	0.1	62
Cabbage, summer	200	0	0.20	0.11	0.03	0.7	0.3	0.09	0	40	0.21	0.1	48
Cabbage, white	40	0	0.20	0.12	0.01	0.3	0.2	0.18	0	34	0.21	0.1	35
(The amount of carotene in leafy vegetables depends on the amount of chlorophyll, and the outer green leaves may contain 50 times as much as inner white ones. This is the value for inner leaves. Outer leaves contain -tocopherol per 100 g/4 oz)													
Carrots, old	11764	0	0.09	0.13	0.01	0.2	0.2	0.06	0	8	0.27	0.3	2
Carrots, young	7807	0	0.56	0.04	0.02	0.2	0.1	0.07	0	28	0.25	0.6	4
(Levels of carotene in carrots ranged from 4,300 to 11,000 g per 100 g/4 oz.)													
Celery	50	0	0.20	0.06	0.01	0.3	0.1	0.03	0	16	0.40	0.1	8

continued ▶

SPECIFIC
CONDITIONS

Food	Carotene g	Vit D g	Vit E mg	Thiamin mg	Riboflavin mg	Niacin mg	Tryptophan mg	Vit B6 mg	Vit B12 g	Folate g	Pantothenate mg	Biotin g	Vit C mg
Cherries	25	0	0.13	0.03	0.03	0.2	0.1	0.05	0	5	0.26	0.4	11
Cinnamon, ground	177	0	N	0.02	0.04	1.3	N	0.16	0	6	0.36	N	4
Cloves, dried	320	0	N	0.11	0.27	1.5	N	N	0	0	N	N	0
Coconut milk	0	0	Tr	0.03	0.06	0.1	0.1	0.03	0	N	0.04	N	2
Courgette, raw	610	0	N	0.12	0.02	0.3	0.3	0.15	0	52	0.08	N	21
Cranberries	22	0	N	0.03	0.02	0.1	0.1	0.07	0	2	0.22	N	13
Cucumber	74	0	0.04	0.03	0.02	0.2	0.1	0.01	0	14	0.32	0.8	2
(Levels of carotene in cucumber can be as high as 260 g per 100 g/4 oz. In peeled cucumbers, the carotene ranges from 0 to 35 g per 100 g/4 oz.)													
Elderberries	(360)	0	N	0.07	0.07	1.0	0.1	0.24	0	17	0.16	1.8	27
Fennel, Florence	140	0	N	0.06	0.01	0.6	N	0.06	0	42	N	N	5
Garlic	Tr	0	0.01	0.13	0.03	0.3	1.9	0.38	0	5	N	N	17
Ginger, fresh	0	0	0.26	0.02	0.03	0.8	0.2	0.16	0.0	11	0.20	N	5

Food	Carotene g	Vit D g	Vit E mg	Thiamin mg	Riboflavin mg	Niacin mg	Tryptophan mg	Vit B6 mg	Vit B12 g	Folate g	Pantothenate mg	Biotin g	Vit C mg
Grapefruit	17	0	(0.19)	0.05	0.02	0.3	0.1	0.03	0	26	0.28	(1.0)	36
(Pink varieties of grapefruit contain approximately 280 g of carotene per 100 g/4 oz.)													
Grapes	17	0	Tr	0.05	0.01	0.2	Tr	0.10	0	2	0.05	0.3	3
Kale, curly	3145	0	(1.70)	0.08	0.09	1.0	0.7	0.26	0	120	0.09	0.5	110
Kiwi fruit	40	0	N	0.01	0.03	0.3	0.3	0.15	0	N	N	N	59
Kohlrabi, boiled in unsalted water	Tr	0	Tr	0.08	0.01	0.2	0.2	0.11	0	47	0.11	N	27
Leeks, boiled in unsalted water	150	0	0.78	0.02	0.02	0.4	0.2	0.05	0	40	0.1	1.0	7
Lemons, whole without pips	18	0	N	0.05	0.04	0.2	0.1	0.11	0	N	0.23	0.5	58
Lettuce, average	60	0	0.64	0.14	0.05	0.5	0.1	0.02	0	60	0.19	0.7	1
Lettuce, butterhead	910	0	0.57	0.15	0.03	0.5	0.1	0.08	0	57	0.18	0.7	7
Lettuce, cos	290	0	0.57	0.12	0.02	0.6	0.1	0.03	0	55	(0.18)	0.7	5
Lettuce, iceberg	50	0	0.57	0.11	0.01	0.3	0.1	0.03	0	53	(0.18)	0.7	3

continued ▶

SPECIFIC
CONDITIONS

Food	Carotene g	Vit D g	Vit E mg	Thiamin mg	Riboflavin mg	Niacin mg	Tryptophan mg	Vit B6 mg	Vit B12 g	Folate g	Pantothenate mg	Biotin g	Vit C mg
Lettuce, Webbs	180	0	0.57	0.11	0.01	0.3	0.1	0.03	0	56	(0.18)	0.7	5
(Carotene in lettuce are average figures. The outer green leaves may contain 50 times as much carotene as the inner white ones.)													
Limes, peeled	12	0	N	0.03	0.02	0.2	0.1	(0.08)	0	8	0.22	N	46
Mangos, ripe	696	0	1.05	0.04	0.05	0.5	1.3	0.13	0	N	0.16	N	37
(Levels of carotene in mangos ranged from 300 to 3,000 g per 100 g/4 oz.)													
Melon, average	N	0	0.10	0.03	0.01	0.4	Tr	0.09	0	3	0.17	N	17
Melon, canteloupe	1000	0	0.10	0.04	0.02	0.6	Tr	0.11	0	5	0.13	N	26
Melon, galia	N	0	(0.10)	(0.03)	(0.01)	(0.4)	Tr	(0.09)	0	(3)	(0.17)	N	15
Melon, honeydew	48	0	0.10	0.03	0.01	0.3	Tr	0.06	0	2	0.21	N	9
Melon, watermelon	116	0	(0.10)	0.05	0.01	0.1	Tr	0.1	0	2	0.21	1.0	8
(The carotene level is an average value. Carotene levels have been reported for rock melons at 835 g and for canteloupe melons at 1,510 to 1,930 g per 100 g/4 oz)													

Food	Carotene µg	Vit D µg	Vit E mg	Thiamin mg	Riboflavin mg	Niacin mg	Tryptophan mg	Vit B6 mg	Vit B12 µg	Folate µg	Pantothenate mg	Biotin µg	Vit C mg
Mint, fresh	740	0	5.00	0.12	0.33	1.1	N	N	0.0	110	N	N	31
Onions	10	0	0.31	0.13	Tr	0.7	0.3	0.20	0	17	0.11	0.9	5
Oranges	55	0	0.35	0.22	0.03	0.5	0.1	0.05	0	33	0.27	1.0	52
Papaya (pawpaw)	810	0	N	0.03	0.04	0.3	0.1	0.03	0	1	0.22	N	60
Parsley	4040	0	1.70	0.23	0.06	1.0	0.5	0.09	0	170	0.30	0.4	190
Parsnip	30	0	1.00	0.23	0.01	1.0	0.5	0.11	0	87	0.50	0.1	17
Peaches	58	0	N	0.02	0.04	0.6	0.2	0.02	0	3	0.17	(0.2)	31
Pears, average	15	0	Tr	0.03	0.04	0.2	0.1	0.04	0	6	0.08	0.3	3
Pears, Comice	15	0	0.50	0.02	0.03	0.2	Tr	0.2	0	2	0.07	0.2	6
Pears, Conference	15	0	0.50	0.02	0.03	0.2	Tr	0.2	0	2	0.07	0.2	6
Pears, William	25	0	0.50	0.02	0.03	0.2	Tr	0.02	0	2	0.07	0.2	6
Pineapple	18	0	0.10	0.08	0.03	0.3	0.1	0.09	0	5	0.16	0.3	12
Plums, average	295	0	0.61	0.05	0.03	1.1	0.1	0.05	0	3	0.15	Tr	4
Prunes	155	0	N	0.10	0.20	1.5	0.5	0.24	0	4	0.46	Tr	Tr
Porridge oats, unfortified	0	0	0.59	1.05	0.05	0.8	2.7	0.34	0	32	0.75	19	0
Potatoes, early new	Tr	0	(0.06)	0.15	0.02	0.4	0.4	(0.44)	0	25	(0.37)	(0.3)	16

continued ▶

SPECIFIC CONDITIONS

139

Food	Carotene μg	Vit D μg	Vit E mg	Thiamin mg	Riboflavin mg	Niacin mg	Tryptophan mg	Vit B6 mg	Vit B12 μg	Folate μg	Pantothenate mg	Biotin μg	Vit C mg
Potatoes, main crop, average (Freshly dug potatoes contain 21 mg of vitamin C per 100 g/4 oz. This falls to 9 mg per 100 g/4 oz after three months' storage and to 7 mg after nine months.)	Tr	0	0.06	0.21	0.01	0.6	0.5	0.06	0	10	0.26	0.3	3
Pumpkin seeds	230	0	N	0.23	0.32	1.7	7.1	N	0	N	N	N	0
Radishes	Tr	0	0	0.03	Tr	0.4	0.1	0.07	0	38	0.18	N	17
Raspberries	6	0	0.48	0.03	0.05	0.5	0.3	0.06	0	33	0.24	1.9	32
Seaweed,(nori, dried)	14910	0	N	0.24	1.34	5.5	N	0.07	27.5	N	N	N	14
Sesame seeds	6	0	2.53	0.93	0.17	5.0	5.4	0.75	0	97	2.14	11	0
Spinach	3535	0	1.71	0.07	0.09	1.2	0.7	0.17	0	150	(0.27)	(0.1)	26
Spring onions (scallions) (bulbs and tops)	620	0	N	0.05	0.03	0.5	0.5	0.13	0	54	0.07	N	26
Strawberries	Tr	0	0.39	0.02	0.02	0.6	0.1	0.03	0	61	0.37	1.2	57
Sunflower seeds	15	0	37.77	1.60	0.19	4.1	5.0	N	0	N	N	N	0
Sweet potato (boiled in unsalted water)	3960	0	0.28	0.07	0.01	0.5	0.3	0.05	0.0	8	0.53	N	17

Food	Carotene g	Vit D g	Vit E mg	Thiamin mg	Riboflavin mg	Niacin mg	Tryptophan mg	Vit B6 mg	Vit B12 g	Folate g	Pantothenate mg	Biotin g	Vit C mg
Tomatoes	349	0	0.52	0.04	0.01	0.6	0.1	0.06	0	23	0.29	1.4	22
Turmeric, ground	15	0	N	0.09	0.11	3.7	N	N	0	0	N	N	0
Turnip	20	0	Tr	0.05	0.01	0.4	0.2	0.08	0	14	0.20	0.1	17
Turnip tops (boiled in unsalted water)	(6000)	0	2.87	0.06	0.20	0.5	0.6	0.18	0	120	0.27	(0.4)	40
Watercress	2520	0	1.46	0.16	0.06	0.3	0.5	0.23	0	45	0.10	0.4	62
Wheatgerm	0	0	16.20	1.8	0.63	6.7	6	2.58	0	277	2.6	23.4	0
Yoghurt, Greek-style, plain	Tr	0.1	0.38	0.12	0.13	0.1	1.0	0.01	0.2	18	0.56	1.5	Tr
Yoghurt, whole milk, plain	21	0	0.05	0.06	0.27	0.2	1.3	0.10	0.2	18	0.50	2.6	1

Minerals

Data relates to quantities per 100 g/4 oz of whole raw fruits or vegetables before being juiced.

Food	Sodium mg	Potassium mg	Calcium mg	Magnesium mg	Phosphorus mg	Iron mg	Copper mg	Zinc mg	Sulphur mg	Chloride mg	Manganese mg	Selenium g	Iodine g
Alfalfa sprouts	6	79	32	27	70	1.0	0.16	0.9	N	N	0.2	N	N
Almonds, flaked and ground	14	780	240	270	550	3.00	1.00	3.2	N	18	1.70	2	2
Apples, cooking, peeled	2	88	4	3	7	0.1	0.02	Tr		N	0.02	Tr	4
Apples, eating, average	3	120	4	5	11	0.1	0.02	0.1	6	Tr	0.1	Tr	Tr
Apples, Cox's Pippin	3	130	4	6	12	0.2	Tr	Tr	6	Tr	Tr	Tr	Tr
Apples, Golden Delicious	4	110	4	5	9	0.2	0.04	0.1	6	Tr	0.1	Tr	Tr

Food	Sodium mg	Potassium mg	Calcium mg	Magnesium mg	Phosphorus mg	Iron mg	Copper mg	Zinc mg	Sulphur mg	Chloride mg	Manganese mg	Selenium g	Iodine g
Apples, Granny Smith	2	120	4	4	9	0.1	0.02	Tr	6	1	0.1	Tr	Tr
Apples, red dessert	1	110	4	5	10	0.1	0.04	Tr	6	Tr	Tr	Tr	Tr
Apricots	2	270	15	11	20	0.5	0.06	0.1	6	3	0.1	(1)	N
Artichoke, Jerusalem (boiled in unsalted water)	3	420	30	11	33	0.4	0.12	0.1	22	58	N	N	N
Asparagus (boiled in unsalted water)	1	220	25	13	50	0.6	0.08	0.7	47	60	0.2	1	Tr
Avocado (average, raw)	6	450	11	25	39	0.40	0.19	0.4	N	6	0.20	Tr	2
Bananas, raw	Tr	330	6	27	23	0.27	0.10	0.2		109	0.36	Tr	3
Basil, fresh	9	300	250	11	37	5.50	N	0.7	N	N	N	N	N
Beans, green or French	Tr	230	36	17	38	1.2	0.01	0.2	17	9	N	N	N

continued ▶

Food	Sodium mg	Potassium mg	Calcium mg	Magnesium mg	Phosphorus mg	Iron mg	Copper mg	Zinc mg	Sulphur mg	Chloride mg	Manganese mg	Selenium µg	Iodine µg
Beansprouts, mung	5	74	20	18	48	1.7	0.08	0.3	N	15	0.3	N	N
Beetroot (red beet)	66	380	20	11	51	1.0	0.02	0.4	16	59	0.7	Tr	N
Blackberries	2	160	41	23	31	0.7	0.11	0.2	9	22	1.4	Tr	N
Blackcurrants	3	370	60	17	43	1.3	0.14	0.3	33	15	0.3	N	N
Blueberries	2	66	10	5	16	0.55	0.06	0.1		53	0.69	Tr	2
Broccoli, green	8	370	56	22	87	1.7	0.02	0.6	130	100	0.2	Tr	2
Brussels sprouts, raw	6	450	26	8	77	0.7	0.02	0.5	93	38	0.2	N	1
Cabbage, average	7	228	56	14	37	0.52	0.04	0.3	N	75	0.18	1	1
Cabbage, Chinese	7	230	54	7	27	0.6	0.02	0.2	N	18	0.3	N	N
Cabbage, January King	3	270	68	6	46	0.6	0.02	0.4	N	45	0.2	(2)	2
Cabbage, red	8	250	60	9	37	0.4	0.01	0.1	68	45	0.2	(2)	(2)
Cabbage, Savoy	5	320	53	7	44	1.1	0.03	0.3	88	48	0.2	(2)	2

Food	Sodium mg	Potassium mg	Calcium mg	Magnesium mg	Phosphorus mg	Iron mg	Copper mg	Zinc mg	Sulphur mg	Chloride mg	Manganese mg	Selenium g	Iodine g
Cabbage, summer	7	240	38	12	35	0.4	0.01	0.1	N	14	0.2	(2)	2
Cabbage, white	7	240	49	6	29	0.5	0.01	0.2	54	40	0.2	Tr	2
Carrots, old	27	178	26	7	16	0.23	0.03	0.1	7	122	0.07	Tr	Tr
Carrots, young	40	240	34	9	25	0.4	0.02	0.2	(7)	39	(0.1)	(1)	(2)
Celery	60	320	41	5	21	0.4	0.01	0.1	15	130	0.1	(3)	N
Cherries	1	210	13	10	21	0.2	0.07	0.1	7	Tr	0.1	(1)	Tr
Cinnamon, ground	10	431	1002	60	64	8.32	0.34	1.8	N	N	17.47	3	N
Cloves	240	1100	730	260	110	5.6	0.49	2.2	N	N	8.5	N	N
Coconut milk	110	280	29	30	30	0.10	0.04	0.1	N	180	N	N	N
Courgette, raw	1	360	25	22	45	0.80	0.02	0.3	N	45	0.10	1	N
Cucumber	3	140	18	8	49	0.3	0.01	0.1	11	17	0.1	Tr	3
Cranberries	2	95	12	7	11	0.7	0.05	0.2	11	Tr	0.1	Tr	N
Elderberries	1	290	37	0	48	1.6	N	N	N	N	N	N	N
Fennel, Florence	11	440	24	8	26	0.3	0.02	0.5	N	27	N	N	N

continued ▶

Food	Sodium mg	Potassium mg	Calcium mg	Magnesium mg	Phosphorus mg	Iron mg	Copper mg	Zinc mg	Sulphur mg	Chloride mg	Manganese mg	Selenium g	Iodine g
Garlic	4	620	19	25	170	1.9	0.06	1.0	N	73	0.5	2	3
Ginger, fresh	13	415	16	43	34	0.60	0.23	0.3	N	N	0.23	N	N
Grapes, average	1	215	10	7	19	0.23	0.09	Tr	8	54	0.06	Tr	1
Grapefruit	3	200	23	9	20	0.1	0.02	Tr	7	3	Tr	(1)	N
Kale, curly	43	450	130	34	61	1.7	0.03	0.4	N	68	0.8	(2)	N
Kiwi fruit	4	290	25	15	32	0.4	0.13	0.1	16	39	0.1	N	N
Kohlrabi	4	340	30	10	35	0.3	Tr	0.1	N	34	0.1	N	1
Leeks	2	260	24	3	44	1.1	0.02	0.2	58	59	0.2	(1)	N
Lemons, whole without pips	5	150	85	12	18	0.5	0.26	0.1	12	5	N	(1)	N
Lettuce, average	3	220	28	6	28	0.7	0.01	0.2	16	47	0.3	(1)	2
Lettuce, butterhead	5	360	53	8	43	1.5	0.04	0.4	16	67	0.3	(1)	2
Lettuce, cos	1	220	21	6	29	0.6	Tr	0.2	16	48	0.3	(1)	2
Lettuce, iceberg	2	160	19	5	18	0.4	0.01	0.1	16	42	0.3	(1)	2

Food	Sodium mg	Potassium mg	Calcium mg	Magnesium mg	Phosphorus mg	Iron mg	Copper mg	Zinc mg	Sulphur mg	Chloride mg	Manganese mg	Selenium g	Iodine g
Lettuce, Webbs	4	150	20	5	21	0.5	0.01	0.1	16	29	0.3	(1)	2
Limes, peeled	2	130	23	11	18	0.4	0.05	0.1	N	N	Tr	N	N
Mangos, ripe	2	180	12	13	16	0.7	0.12	0.1	N	N	0.3	N	N
Melon, average	24	190	14	11	13	0.2	Tr	Tr	9	55	Tr	Tr	N
Melon, canteloupe	8	210	20	11	13	0.3	Tr	Tr	12	44	Tr	Tr	(4)
Melon, galia	31	150	13	12	10	0.2	Tr	0.1	9	75	Tr	Tr	N
Melon, honeydew	32	210	9	10	16	0.1	Tr	Tr	6	45	Tr	Tr	N
Melon, watermelon	2	100	7	8	9	0.3	0.03	0.2	N	N	Tr	Tr	Tr
Mint, fresh	15	260	210	N	75	9.50	N	N	N	34	1.40	N	N
Onions	3	160	25	4	30	0.3	0.05	0.2	51	25	0.1	(1)	3
Oranges	1	122	24	8	16	0.11	0.03	Tr	10	73	0.02	Tr	1
Papaya (pawpaw), raw	5	200	23	11	13	0.5	0.08	0.2	13	11	0.1	N	N

continued ▶

SPECIFIC CONDITIONS

147

Food	Sodium mg	Potassium mg	Calcium mg	Magnesium mg	Phosphorus mg	Iron mg	Copper mg	Zinc mg	Sulphur mg	Chloride mg	Manganese mg	Selenium g	Iodine g
Parsley	33	760	200	23	64	7.7	0.03	0.7	N	160	0.2	(1)	N
Parsnip	10	450	41	23	74	0.6	0.05	0.3	17	49	0.5	2	N
Peaches, raw	1	160	7	9	22	0.4	0.06	0.1	6	Tr	0.1	(1)	3
Pears, average	3	150	11	7	13	0.2	0.06	0.1	5	1	Tr	Tr	1
Pears, Comice	3	150	12	7	13	0.2	0.04	0.1	5	Tr	Tr	Tr	1
Pears, Conference	4	150	11	7	13	0.2	0.06	0.1	5	2	Tr	Tr	1
Pears, William	2	150	9	8	12	0.1	0.08	0.2	5	1	0.1	Tr	1
Pineapple, raw	2	160	18	16	10	0.2	0.11	0.1	3	29	0.5	Tr	Tr
Plums, average	2	240	13	8	23	0.4	0.10	0.1	5	Tr	0.1	Tr	Tr
Porridge oats, unfortified	1	372	50	114	387	3.64	0.37	2.3	N	87	3.66	3	Tr
Potatoes, new (boiled in unsalted water)	3	377	11	18	44	0.61	0.08	0.20	(30)	88	0.12	Tr	Tr

Food	Sodium mg	Potassium mg	Calcium mg	Magnesium mg	Phosphorus mg	Iron mg	Copper mg	Zinc mg	Sulphur mg	Chloride mg	Manganese mg	Selenium g	Iodine g
Potatoes, main crop	7	360	5	17	37	0.4	0.08	0.3	30	66	0.1	1	3
Prunes	12	860	38	27	83	2.9	0.16	0.5	19	3	0.3	3	N
Pumpkin seeds	18	820	39	270	850	10	1.57	6.6	N	N	N	6	N
Radishes, red	11	240	19	5	20	0.6	0.01	0.2	38	37	0.1	(2)	(1)
Raspberries	3	170	25	19	31	0.7	0.10	0.3	17	22	0.4	N	N
Seaweed, (nori, dried)	790	2840	430	12	350	19.60	1.60	6.4	N	N	6.00	N	1470
Sesame seeds	20	570	670	370	720	10.40	1.46	5.3	N	10	1.50	N	N
Spinach mature, raw	140	500	170	54	45	2.1	0.04	0.7	20	98	0.6	(1)	2
Spring onions (scallions) (bulbs and tops)	7	260	39	12	29	1.9	0.06	0.4	(50)	31	0.2	N	N
Strawberries	1	170	17	12	26	0.25	0.03	0.1	13	62	0.31	Tr	1
Sunflower seeds	3	730	110	400	660	6.60	2.35	5.3	N	N	2.30	51	N

continued ▶

SPECIFIC
CONDITIONS

Food	Sodium mg	Potassium mg	Calcium mg	Magnesium mg	Phosphorus mg	Iron mg	Copper mg	Zinc mg	Sulphur mg	Chloride mg	Manganese mg	Selenium g	Iodine g
Sweet potato (boiled in unsalted water)	40	300	23	45	50	0.70	0.14	0.3	N	65	0.40	1	2
Tomatoes, standard, raw	2	223	8	8,	22	0.24	0.03	0.1	11	84	0.12	Tr	2
Turmeric, ground	31	2910	170	190	290	39.50	1.00	3.2	N	N	3.70	N	N
Turnip	15	280	48	8	41	0.2	0.01	0.1	22	39	0.1	(1)	N
Turnips tops (boiled in unsalted water)	7	78	98	10	45	3.1	0.09	0.4	39	15	N	N	N
Watercress	49	230	170	15	52	2.2	0.01	0.7	100	170	0.6	N	N
Wheatgerm	3	1045	45	240	1047	8.08	0.82	14	N	107	13.5	18	Tr
Yoghurt, Greek-style, plain	66	184	126	13	138	0.11	Tr	0.5	N	159	Tr	3	39
Yoghurt, whole milk, plain	80	280	200	19	170	0.10	Tr	0.7	N	170	Tr	2	63

Useful addresses

Planet Organic Ltd

42 Westbourne Grove
London
W2 5SH
Tel: 020 7221 1345 email talktous@planetorganic.com
www.planetorganic.com

Specialist Herbal Supplies

(suppliers of wheatgrass in powder and capsule form)

Portslade Hall
18 Station Road
Portslade
East Sussex
BN41 1GB
Tel: 01273 424333 email: sales@shs100.com
www.shs100.com

NutriCentre

(suppliers of healthcare products)

Unit 3 Kendal Court
Kendal Avenue
London
W3 0RU
Tel: 0345 2222 828 email: enquiry@nutricentre.com
www.nutricentre.com

BioCare® Ltd

Lakeside
180 Lifford Lane
Kings Norton
Birmingham
B30 3NU
Tel: 0121 433 3727 email: customerservice@biocare.co.uk
www.biocare.co.uk

The Fresh Network

Unit 4 Aylsham Business Estate
Shepheards Close
Aylsham
Norfolk
NR11 6SZ
Tel: 01263 738 661 email: info@fresh-network.com
www.fresh-network.com

Bibliography

Amazing Claims for Chlorophyll (Lowell), Nutrition Forum, 7/87.

Stephen Barrett, Dietary Supplements: Appropriate Use, Quackwatch website, 1999.

Stephen Barrett, Juicing, Quackwatch website, 4 September 1999.

Ruth Bircher-Benner, *Eating Your Way to Health*, Faber and Faber, 1961.

Stephen Blauer, *The Juicing Book*, Avery, NY, 1989.

Cherie Calbom & Maureen Keane, *Juicing for Life*, Avery Publishing Group, 1992.

Brian R. Clement and Theresa Foy Digeronimo, *Living Foods for Optimum Health*, Prima Health, 1998.

Vernon Coleman, *Eat Green, Lose Weight*, Angus & Robertson, 1990.

Alan Davidson, *The Oxford Companion of Food*, Oxford University Press, 1999.

Alan Davidson, Charlotte Knox, *Fruit, a Connoisseur's Guide and Cookbook*, Mitchell Beazley, 1991.

John and Lucie Davidson, *A Harmony of Science and Nature*, Holistic Research Co., 1999.

Davidson, Passmore, Brock, Truswell, *Human Nutrition and Dietetics*, 7th edition, Churchill Livingstone, 1979.

Genry and Lynne Devereux, *Juice It Up*, 101 Productions, Santa Rosa, USA.

Finglas P.M., Roe M.A., Pinchen H.M., Berry R., Church S.M., Dodhia S.K., Farron-Wilson M. & Swan G. (2014) McCance and Widdowson's *The Composition of Foods*, 7th summary edition. Cambridge: Royal Society of Chemistry.

Dr Bernard Jensen, *Juicing Therapy*, Escondido, 1992.

Leslie Kenton with Russell Cronin, *Juice High*, Ebury Press, 1996.

Leslie Kenton, *Lean Revolution*, Ebury Press, 1994.

Leslie and Susannah Kenton, *Raw Energy*, Arrow, 1984.

Jethro Kloss, *Back to Eden*, Back to Eden Books, revised and expanded 1994.

Jay Kordich, *The Juiceman's Power of Juicing*, William Marrow and Co. Inc., NY, 1992.

William H. Lee, *The Book of Raw Fruit, Vegetable Juices and Drinks*, Keats, Conn., 1982.

William H. Lee, *Getting the Best out of Your Juicer*, Keats, Conn., 1992.

Barry Lynch, *BBC Health Check*, BBC Books, 1989.

Leonard Mervyn, *Vitamins A, D and K*, Thorsons, 1984.

Morse, Rivers, Heughan, Barrie and Jenkins, *The Family Guide to Food and Health*, 1988.

National Council Against Health Fraud, Wheatgrass Therapy: C.1994, www.ncahf.org.

J.O. Rodale, *The Complete Book of Food and Nutrition*, Rodale Books Inc., Pennsylvania, 1972.

Jo Rogers, *The Encyclopedia of Food and Nutrition*, Merehurst, 1990.

Tom Sanders and Peter Bazalgette, *The Food Revolution*, Bantam Press, 1991.

Briony Thomas, *The Manual of Dietetic Practice*, edited by the British Dietetic Association, Blackwell Scientific Publications, 1988.

Thorson's Editorial Board, *The Complete Raw Juice Therapy*, Thorson, 1989.

Michael van Straten and Barbara Griggs, *Superfoods*, Dorling Kindersley, 1990.

N.W. Walker, *Become Younger*, Norwalk Press, Arizona, revised 1995.

N.W. Walker, *Colon Health: The Key to Vibrant Life*, Norwalk Press, Arizona, 1979.

N.W. Walker, *Diet and Salad*, Norwalk Press, Arizona, 1986.

N.W. Walker, *Fresh Vegetable and Fruit Juices*, Norwalk Press, Arizona, 1978.

N.W. Walker, *The Natural Way to Vibrant Health*, Norwalk Press, Arizona, 1995.

What the Heck is Essiac, http://.members.oal.com/essiac/indexhtn.

Caroline Wheater, *Beta Carotene: How It Can Help You to Better Health*, Thorsons, 1991.

Caroline Wheater, *The Juicing Detox Diet*, Thorsons, 1993.

Caroline Wheater, *Juicing for Health*, Thorsons, 1993.

Ann Wigmore, *The Wheatgrass Book*, Avery Publishing Group Inc., Wayne, New Jersey, 1985.

Judith Wills, *Slim and Healthy Mediterranean*, Conran Octopus, 1992.

Index